Pediatric Anesthesia Practice

Edited by

RONALD S. LITMAN, D. O., F. A. A. P.

Associate Professor of Anesthesiology & Pediatrics
University of Pennsylvania School of Medicine
Philadelphia, PA
Director of Clinical Research
Division of General Anesthesia
Department of Anesthesiology and Critical Care
The Children's Hospital of Philadelphia

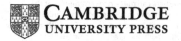

CAMBRIDGE
UNIVERSITY PRESS

CAMBRIDGE
UNIVERSITY PRESS

32 Avenue of the Americas, New York NY 10013-2473, USA

Cambridge University Press is part of the University of Cambridge.

It furthers the University's mission by disseminating knowledge in the pursuit of education, learning and research at the highest international levels of excellence.

www.cambridge.org
Information on this title: www.cambridge.org/9780521709378

© 2007, 2003 Pediatric Anesthesia Practice by PocketMedicine.com, Inc.

First published 2007

A catalogue record for this publication is available from the British Library

Library of Congress Cataloguing in Publication data

Litman, Ronald S.
Pediatric anesthesia practice / Ronald Litman.
    p.   cm.
ISBN-13: 978-0-521-70937-8 (pbk.)
ISBN-10: 0-521-70937-7 (pbk.)
1. Pediatric anesthesia.   I. Title.
[DNLM: 1. Anesthesia –methods.   2. Pediatrics –methods.   3. Child.
WO 440 L776p 2007]
RD139.L58   2007
617'.6083 – dc22   2007016727

ISBN 978-0-521-70937-8 Paperback

. . . .

NOTICE

Because of the dynamic nature of medical practice and drug selection and dosage, users are advised that decisions regarding drug therapy must be based on the independent judgment of the clinician, changing information about a drug (e.g., as reflected in the literature and manufacturer's most current product information), and changing medical practices.

While great care has been taken to ensure the accuracy of the information presented, users are advised that the authors, editors, contributors, and publisher make no warranty, express or implied, with respect to, and are not responsible for, the currency, completeness, or accuracy of the information contained in this publication, nor for any errors, omissions, or the application of this information, nor for any consequences arising therefrom. Users are encouraged to confirm the information contained herein with other sources deemed authoritative. Ultimately, it is the responsibility of the treating physician, relying on experience and knowledge of the patient, to determine dosages and the best treatment for the patient. Therefore, the author(s), editors, contributors, and the publisher make no warranty, express or implied, and shall have no liability to any person or entity with regard to claims, loss, or damage caused, or alleged to be caused, directly or indirectly, by the use of information contained in this publication.

Further, the author(s), editors, contributors, and the publisher are not responsible for misuse of any of the information provided in this publication, for negligence by the user, or for any typographical errors.

Contents

PART TWO. SURGICAL PROCEDURES

PART THREE. REGIONAL ANESTHESIA

Preface

The care of children in the perianesthetic period requires a unique knowledge base and skill set that differs widely from that required for the anesthetic care of the adult patient. The physiology of organ systems is developing throughout childhood, and thus, anesthetic pharmacology differs correspondingly. Infancy and childhood are associated with a myriad of medical problems that often carry into adolescence and adulthood. For these reasons, anesthesiology residents and anesthesia practitioners who are not experts in pediatric anesthesia require a complete and accurate guide to providing care that is consistent with the standards implemented at the leading children's hospitals. *Pediatric Anesthesia Practice* aims to provide such a point-of-care guide, utilizing contributions by 61 authors from institutions throughout the world, and edited in a uniform style.

This text is organized into three main sections: Surgical Procedures, Coexisting Diseases, and Regional Anesthesia. The Surgical Procedures section contains details on the anesthetic management of more than 100 common pediatric surgical procedures. Each is divided into six separate important sections that cover the entire perioperative period. These include the common coexisting diseases associated with that particular procedure, preoperative assessment strategies, procedural considerations, anesthetic plan recommendations, pain management strategies, and postoperative considerations.

The section on Coexisting Diseases contains chapters encompassing the most common and most important pediatric diseases with anesthetic implications. Each chapter is divided into four main sections that include information on the aspects of that particular disease, preoperative assessment of patients with that disease, intraoperative management of those patients, and postoperative considerations.

The section on Regional Anesthesia contains chapters with details on the most commonly performed pediatric regional anesthesia techniques. Each chapter contains four separate subsections on indications for the technique, pre-procedural assessment of the patient, procedural management of the technique, and postoperative considerations of the technique.

Pediatric Anesthesia Practice is, I believe, an indispensable resource for a variety of different anesthesia practitioners that provide anesthesia care to children.

Ronald S. Litman

PART ONE

Coexisting Diseases

ANTERIOR MEDIASTINAL MASS

PAUL STRICKER, MD

BACKGROUND
- Most common cause: lymphoma
- Suspect in pts presenting for cervical mass biopsy.
- Other dxs: neuroblastoma, teratoma, germ cell tumor, bronchogenic cyst, foregut cyst, lymphangioma, mesenchymal tumor
- Symptoms due to compression of anatomic structures
- Symptoms worse when supine
- Symptoms may be relieved by lateral or upright position.
- Clinical: cough, hoarseness, dyspnea, wheezing, orthopnea, stridor, chest pain, syncope, SVC syndrome, tracheal deviation, retractions
- Asymptomatic or nonspecific: fever, fatigue, weight loss

PREOPERATIVE ASSESSMENT
- Preoperative radiation tx may interfere with accurate histologic dx & optimal tx regimens.
- Physical exam: orthopnea, tracheal deviation, jugular venous distention, wheezing, retractions, unilateral decreased breath sounds
- CXR: tracheal deviation, tracheal compression, abnormal cardiothymic silhouette
- Echo: direct compression of cardiac chambers and/or great vessels, pericardial effusion
- CT: assess severity & location of tracheal compression
- Preop sedation: avoid or give in monitored setting
- Antisialagogue (e.g., glycopyrrolate) useful

- Obtain IV access prior to OR, ideally in lower extremity.
- Correct preexisting dehydration or hypovolemia.

INTRAOPERATIVE MANAGEMENT
- Potential catastrophic airway or cardiovascular collapse during induction of anesthesia
- Monitors: std; A-line for great vessel or cardiac compression
- All sized endotracheal tubes and rigid bronch immed avail in OR
- For severe cases, ECMO or CPB stand-by
- Liberal fluid administration if great vessel/cardiac compression
- Position: semi-recumbent, sitting, or lateral
- Local anesthesia without sedation is safest strategy, but not feasible for small children.
- Most important to avoid airway/CV collapse: MAINTAIN SPONTANEOUS VENTILATION
- Mask or LMA OK
- Ketamine allows spontaneous ventilation & provides sympathetic stimulation.
- Sevoflurane or IV agents OK if titrated to avoid apnea
- Paralysis & controlled ventilation OK for mild cases, but no way to predict safety
- Tx of airway obstruction: positive pressure, change position to lateral, sitting or prone if CV arrest
- Rigid bronch may bypass airway obstruction.
- ECMO or CPB as lifesaving measure

POSTOPERATIVE CONCERNS
- Airway obstruction may occur postop during recovery.
- Recover in lateral or semi-recumbent position.
- Titrate opioids: avoid apnea.

ASTHMA

SANJAY M. BHANANKER, MD, FRCA

BACKGROUND
- Incidence: 7–19%
- Cause: chronic inflammation & mucus hypersecretion of lower airways
- Symptoms: airway hyperreactivity with variable degrees of airflow obstruction
- Strong association with atopy and allergy

PREOPERATIVE ASSESSMENT
- Note severity and frequency of acute exacerbations, precipitating factors.
- Elicit history of drug therapy, especially systemic steroids, to gauge severity.
- If acute exacerbation or URI within 6 wks, consider postponing elective surgery.
- Premed: inhaled beta-2 agonist, steroids (daily meds)
- Anxiolysis with oral midazolam; fear, stress, excitement, or hyperventilation can provoke acute attack

INTRAOPERATIVE MANAGEMENT
- Mask induction with sevoflurane or IV induction with propofol or ketamine
- Minimize airway manipulation.
- Face mask or LMA preferred
- Avoid histamine-releasing drugs: thiopental, morphine, mivacurium, succinylcholine.
- All volatile anesthetic drugs, propofol and ketamine are bronchodilators.
- Administer stress dose of IV hydrocortisone if pt on oral prednisone.

- If intraoperative wheezing occurs:
  - i. Rule out kinked ET tube or bronchial intubation
  - ii. Give 100% oxygen, deepen anesthesia with propofol, ketamine, or volatile agents
  - iii. IV lidocaine 0.5–1 mg/kg bolus
  - iv. Use low respiratory rate and long expiratory time to avoid intrinsic PEEP
  - v. Nebulized beta-2 agonist such as albuterol via ET tube or LMA

POSTOPERATIVE CONCERNS
- Deep extubation for pts with uncomplicated airway avoids risk of bronchospasm during emergence.
- If awake extubation planned, nebulized prophylactic beta-2 agonist, IV lidocaine
- Humidify supplemental oxygen, ensure adequate systemic hydration: dry anesthetic gases and O_2 are potential triggers for asthma.

ATRIAL SEPTAL DEFECT (ASD)

LUIS M. ZABALA, MD

DISEASE CHARACTERISTICS
- Definition: opening in the atrial septum except patent foramen ovale (PFO)
- 7–10% of all CHD
- Incidence of PFO in adults: 25%
- Pathophys: extra load on right side of the heart (L to R shunt)
- Magnitude of shunt relates to size of defect, ventricular compliance, & pulmonary artery pressures.
- L to R shunt: RA & RV enlargement
- Pulmonary vascular changes develop from long-standing volume overload.

- Majority of pts are asymptomatic during childhood.
- In adulthood, extra load on RV leads to CHF, failure to thrive, recurrent respiratory infections, & symptomatic supraventricular dysrhythmias.
- Pulm htn in up to 13% of nonoperated pts

PREOPERATIVE ASSESSMENT

- CXR: RA & RV enlargement.
- ECG: right or left axis deviation possible; incomplete RBBB from stretch in right bundle of His
- Echo: secundum or primum defect; mitral regurg from anterior leaflet cleft.
- Ventricular dysfunction possible from long-standing volume overload
- Cardiology consultation for symptomatic pts
- Premed: PO midazolam (0.5 mg/kg) or PO pentobarbital (4 mg/kg)
- Caution with oversedation & hypoventilation: can worsen PVR & RV fn

INTRAOPERATIVE MANAGEMENT

- Std monitors during noncardiac surgery or transcatheter closure of ASD
- Symptomatic or complicated pts may require additional monitoring.
- Intracardiac surgical repair requires extracorporeal circulation and arterial invasive monitoring.
- Central venous monitoring at discretion of anesthesiologist
- Transesophageal echo helpful to assess de-airing of left heart & adequacy of surgical repair
- Inhalation induction generally safe
- Inhalation agents, narcotics, muscle relaxants, and/or regional anesthesia usually well tolerated
- De-bubble all IV lines.
- Atrial dysrhythmias common in adult unrepaired pt

POSTOPERATIVE CONCERNS

- Immediate or early tracheal extubation possible following uncomplicated surgical repair of ASD
- Pts with good ventricular function prior to repair do not require inotropic support.
- Dopamine 3–5 mcg/kg/min usually sufficient for ventricular dysfunction
- Pulm htn may occur in older pts after ASD repair; use aggressive ventilation & milrinone.
- Pts with unrepaired ASD undergoing noncardiac surgery should be monitored closely for CHF due to volume overload or atrial dysrhythmias.
- Titrate analgesia to pain control without vent depression.

CEREBRAL PALSY

NATHALIA JIMENEZ, MD, MPH

BACKGROUND

- Definition: static motor encephalopathy
- Secondary to perinatal or early childhood (<2 yr) CNS injury
- Incidence 2.4 per 1,000 live births
- 4 categories: spastic (quadriplegia, diplegia, hemiplegia), dyskinetic (dystonia, athetosis, chorea), ataxic (tremor, loss of balance, speech involvement), mixed
- Assoc with developmental delay, visual & cognitive abnormalities, & motor problems possible with normal cognitive function
- Require multiple surgeries: mainly orthopedic (spinal fusion and release of limb contractures)
- Bulbar motor dysfunction predisposes to GE reflux, swallowing disorders & loss of airway protective mechanisms leading to chronic aspiration, recurrent pneumonia, hyperactive airways

- Seizures in 30%: continue anticonvulsant on day of surgery & reinstitute early in postop period
- Baclofen used for muscle spasms, can cause urinary retention & leg weakness
- Abrupt baclofen withdrawal may cause seizures; overdose assoc with decreased consciousness & hypotension

PREOPERATIVE ASSESSMENT
- Premedication tolerated in most pts; reduce dose or avoid if hypotonic
- Anticholinergic will decrease secretions in pts with bulbar dysfunction.

INTRAOPERATIVE MANAGEMENT
- Contractures make positioning and IV access difficult.
- Impaired temp regulation due to hypothalamic dysfunction
- Monitor temperature and use warming measures.
- Inhalation induction safe unless severe reflux
- Increased sensitivity of succinylcholine: use only in emergency situations
- Decreased sensitivity to non-depolarizing muscle relaxants: requires higher doses
- Increased sensitivity to inhaled anesthetics and opioids: use lower doses
- Awake extubation in OR

POSTOPERATIVE CONCERNS
- Pain assessment difficult due to inability to communicate: use modified behavioral pain scales
- Regional techniques for postop analgesia recommended
- Low-dose benzodiazepines (diazepam) to prevent/treat muscle spasms

COARCTATION OF THE AORTA

SCOTT D. MARKOWITZ, MD

BACKGROUND

- Prevalence: 8% of pts with CHD
- Coexisting bicuspid aortic valve, arch hypoplasia, other heart defects
- Hypertension is usually present pre-repair and may persist postop.
- May be repaired with balloon dilation or surgical correction end-to-end anastomosis or subclavian flap arterioplasty
- Residual or recurrent coarct may occur early or late: eval by right arm vs. leg BP & Doppler echo.

PREOPERATIVE ASSESSMENT

- ECG & echo: ventricular hypertrophy/dysfunction, valve dysfunction, residual coarct
- BP measurements in all extremities, identification of previous recurrent laryngeal nerve injury
- Antihypertensive regimen assessed and instructions for day of surgery medication administration given

INTRAOPERATIVE MANAGEMENT

- SBE prophylaxis even after repair
- If pre-repair: BP monitoring on pre-coarct artery (usually right arm except in cases of aberrant subclavian artery)
- If post-repair: monitors accurate in any extremity, except if residual coarct
- Left arm BP unreliable after subclavian flap repair
- Caution with intercostal blocks if intercostal arteries dilated

POSTOPERATIVE CONSIDERATIONS
- Std pain management: opioids & NSAIDs
- Monitor for arrhythmias; resume antihypertensive therapy as appropriate.

CRANIOFACIAL SYNDROMES

SALLY E. RAMPERSAD, MB FRCA

BACKGROUND
- Premature fusion of one or more skull sutures
- Major component of several congenital syndromes: Crouzon, Saethe-Chotzen, Pfeiffer, Carpenter, Aperts

PREOPERATIVE ASSESSMENT
- Previous anesthetic records: airway issues & management
- Examine for obstructing mass (cystic hygroma, large tongue in Beckwith-Wiedemann syndrome; micrognathia/retrognathia in Pierre Robin); limited mouth opening, limited neck mobility, facial asymmetry (Goldenhars).
- Abnl ear form & position indicate other facial anomalies.
- Inform family of potential airway complications.
- Snoring, daytime somnolence, or hx of stridor may indicate significant airway obstruction.
- Cleft lip/palate are part of other syndromes (eg, CHARGE, trisomy 18, velocardiofacial syndrome).
- Associated anomalies: ear, renal, CV
- Avoid pre-op sedation in pts with potential airway obstruction, or administer with anesthesiologist present.
- PO or IV atropine (0.02 mg/kg) as antisialagogue/vagolytic
- Prepare different sizes of facemasks (air-filled cushion for asymmetric face), LMAs, oral & naso-pharyngeal airways, endotracheal tubes, fiberoptic bronchoscopes, stylets.

INTRAOPERATIVE MANAGEMENT

- Need assistance to position & maintain in "sniffing" position
- Oxyscope allows delivery of oxygen during laryngoscopy.
- If airway involvement severe, equipment & personnel for emergency cricothyrotomy or tracheostomy available before induction
- Tracheostomy possible in pts with midface & mandibular abnormalities (Treacher Collins)
- Consider awake laryngoscopy in infants <6 wks or older cooperative child.
- Inhalational induction usually needed for young or developmentally delayed child
- CPAP helpful to overcome airway obstruction as anesthesia deepened
- Demonstrate mask ventilation prior to muscle relaxants.
- Craniectomy carries risk for rapid intraop blood loss and/or venous air embolism (Doppler monitoring can detect); appropriate IV access obtained & blood immediately available.
- Massive blood transfusion occasionally required in craniofacial surgeries; may result in hypothermia, hyperkalemia, coagulopathy, acidosis
- SBE prophylaxis needed for pts with cardiac disease
- Remove throat pack at end of case.
- Extubation when fully awake

POSTOPERATIVE CONCERNS

- Tongue may cause airway obstruction after palate closure.
- Pts with preop airway obstruction at continued postop risk; may need ICU admission
- Blood glucose monitored closely in neonates, especially those with Beckwith-Wiedemann syndrome

CYSTIC FIBROSIS

INGE FALK VAN ROOYEN, MBChB

DISEASE CHARACTERISTICS
- Prevalence: 1:3,000
- Incidence: 20,000 per year
- Most common lethal inherited disorder
- Autosomal recessive disorder of CFTR gene
- Exocrine secretory glands secrete abnormally thick mucus.
- Clinical presentation: recurrent lower respiratory tract infections, coughing, sinus drainage, malnutrition, bronchiectasis, clubbing, cyanosis
- Common surgical procedures: placement of indwelling venous catheter, & nasal polyp resection
- May require lung transplant

PREOPERATIVE ASSESSMENT
- Pulmonary function studies, CXR; consider: ABG, electrolytes, blood glucose, LFTs, ECG
- Premeds: bronchodilators, antibiotics, cardiotonic drugs
- Chest physiotherapy

INTRAOPERATIVE MANAGEMENT
- Inhalational induction may cause excessive coughing; IV induction is usually smoother.
- Airway suctioning, gas humidification helpful
- Avoid dehydration (mucous plugging) and overhydration (excess secretions).
- Intraoperative concerns: pneumothorax; glucose & electrolyte disturbances, cor pulmonale (in end-stage disease)
- Local/regional anesthesia to minimize opiate use & resp depression

■ Awake extubation after ETT suction, lung inflation, & chest physiotherapy

POSTOPERATIVE CONCERNS
■ Encourage coughing, deep breathing and early activity.
■ Plan chest physiotherapy early.
■ Minimize opiates if possible.

EMERGENCE AGITATION

JEFFREY L. GALINKIN, MD

BACKGROUND
■ Most common age group: 9 mos to 6 yrs
■ Occurs during early emergence, 0–30 min after general anesthesia
■ Pts unable to be consoled, controlled, or focus attention
■ Pts disoriented & unaware of surroundings
■ Self-limiting; resolves after sleeping for about 1 hour
■ Upsetting for parents & staff
■ Can cause injury to child, parents, or staff
■ Not linked with postop maladaptive behavior
■ Can occur after any procedure; ultra-short procedures have highest incidence
■ Most common with fast-onset, fast-offset agents (sevoflurane, desflurane)

PREOPERATIVE ASSESSMENT
■ Preop anxiety associated with higher incidence
■ Midazolam premed not associated with higher incidence

INTRAOPERATIVE MANAGEMENT
■ Ketamine, atropine, droperidol, & scopolamine may increase incidence.
■ Lower incidence with propofol anesthetic

- IV opioids and ketorolac decrease incidence from decreased pain.
- Intranasal fentanyl 2 mcg/kg decreases incidence to 2% after myringotomy & tubes.

POSTOPERATIVE MANAGEMENT
- Procedural pain associated with higher incidence
- Child-life programs may decrease anxiety and incidence of EA
- Tx: rule out important causes of agitation (hypoxia, pain)
- Tx: quiet, low-lighted area in PACU conducive to sleep
- Last resort tx: IV fentanyl 1–2 mcg/kg
- Parental or staff comfort rarely effective
- Physical restraints may be necessary until calm.

ENDOCARDIAL CUSHION DEFECTS (ATRIOVENTRICULAR SEPTAL DEFECTS; AVSD)

LUIS M. ZABALA, MD

BACKGROUND
- 5% of all CHD
- Complete AVSD septal defect: interatrial & interventricular components; common AV valve that connects both atria to ventricle
- Transitional AVSD: anterior & posterior bridging leaflets fused above ventricular septum; form distinct mitral & tricuspid components
- Partial AVSD = ostium primum defect: cleft or commissure in left-sided AV valve with 2 functionally distinct AV valve orifices
- Associated with trisomy 21, asplenia or polysplenia syndrome, DiGeorge & Ellis-van Creveld syndrome
- Direction of blood flow through centrally located defects depends on pressures & compliance in all 4 heart chambers and ratio of PVR to SVR.

- Clinical signs in neonate: murmur, possible mild hypoxemia due to intracardiac admixture
- Clinical S&S in children: cardiac failure, failure to thrive, repeated resp infections from increased pulmonary blood flow, increased PA pressure & common AV valve insufficiency

PREOPERATIVE ASSESSMENT
- CXR: RA, RV, LV, PA enlargement
- ECG: superior QRS axis, right & left ventricular hypertrophy, RBBB, variable degrees of AV block
- Complete heart block often seen after surgical repair of AVSD; requires permanent pacemaker
- Echo: crossing AV valve attachments, AV regurgitation, associated intracardiac anomalies
- Cardiology consult for dx of ventricular dysfunction & shunt-induced pulm htn
- Premed: PO midazolam (0.5 mg/kg) or PO pentobarbital (4 mg/kg)
- SBE prophylaxis

INTRAOPERATIVE MANAGEMENT
- Monitoring: guided by severity of disease & complexity of surgical procedure
- IV & inhalation induction usually well tolerated
- In unrepaired children, balance ratio between PVR & SVR by manipulating FiO2 & ventilation.
- Inotropic support & inhaled NO warranted during noncardiac surgery for pts with uncorrected AVSD & residual defects following correction
- Aggressive de-bubbling of IV lines

POSTOPERATIVE CONCERNS
- Titrate analgesia to avoid ventilatory depression and increased PVR.

■ ICU admission for pts with unrepaired defects & postop signs of CHF, ventricular dysfunction, atrial or ventricular dysrhythmias, & oxygen desaturation

---

EX-PREMATURE INFANT

KHA M. TRAN, MD

BACKGROUND

■ Premature = <37 wks gestation
■ Postmenstrual age (wks) = gestational age at birth + chronological age
■ Postconceptional age (wks) = postmenstrual age – 2 weeks
■ Residual apnea of prematurity: home monitoring or caffeine therapy
■ Airway stenosis: tracheostomy size and type, home ventilator, prior ETT sizes
■ Intraventricular hemorrhage: residual neuro deficit, ventriculo-peritoneal shunt
■ Seizures: type, frequency, ketogenic diet, medications, drug levels
■ Cerebral palsy: level of function, flexion or extension contractures
■ Chronic lung disease/bronchopulmonary dysplasia: home oxygen, ventilator, bronchodilators, diuretics
■ Pulmonary hypertension: recent echo, ECG, sildenafil
■ Pulmonary function improves with age, but subtle differences persist into adulthood.
■ Anemia: physiologic or chronic disease
■ Gastroesophageal reflux (GER): medication controlled or need for Nissen fundoplication
■ Failure to thrive: malabsorption, malnutrition, hypoalbuminemia, coagulopathy

- Other congenital anomalies/syndromes: check hx of airway & metabolic management

PREOPERATIVE ASSESSMENT

- Baseline oxygen saturations may be different than normal child.
- Current weight important for drug dosing
- Preop hematocrit <30% associated with apnea
- Other blood tests as indicated by history and physical (electrolytes if taking diuretics)
- Possible difficult IV access
- If <9 mo, sedative premed usually not needed. If older, use clinical judgment.
- Preop anxiolysis may attenuate bronchoconstriction in BPD.
- Respiratory infections more severe than normal children

INTRAOPERATIVE MANAGEMENT

- Multimodal approach to warming: inc room temp, forced air blanket, hot water mattress, etc.
- Mask induction unless severe GER or full stomach
- Smaller ETTs available; check to ensure adequate tidal volumes can be delivered (~10 cc/kg or good chest rise)
- Leak around ETT should be <30 mmHg if possible.
- Use only enough oxygen to maintain normoxemia.
- Chronic lung disease can manifest as restrictive, obstructive, decreased oxygenating ability, or combination.
- Modify ventilator setting & bronchodilators available.
- Minimize barotrauma/volutrauma with careful ventilator management.
- Normocapnia usually higher than normal mmHg
- Treat BPD bronchoconstriction by deepening anesthesia and PEEP.
- Intraoperative blood glucose checks
- If <6 mo, maintenance infusion of 2.5% or 5% dextrose will prevent hypoglycemia.

- Regional analgesia decreases incidence of postop apnea.
- IV caffeine 10 mg/kg decreases incidence of postop apnea.

POSTOPERATIVE CONCERNS
- Central apnea
- If <55–60 weeks PCA, overnight admission for apnea and pulse oximeter monitoring
- Discharge home after 12 apnea-free hrs.

HEMOPHILIA

RONALD S. LITMAN, DO

BACKGROUND
- X-linked inherited bleeding disorder: only males affected
- Hemophilia A: factor VIII deficiency, 1 in 10,000 males
- Hemophilia B: factor IX deficiency, 1 in 25,000 males
- Some female carriers produce low concentrations of these factors, can predispose to bleeding.
- Adequate clotting usually occurs with 30% of normal factor levels.
- Dx by family hx, or prolonged PTT + decreased factor
- Severe (<1% factor): spontaneous bleeding episodes
- Moderate (1–5% factor): may bleed spontaneously; bleeds excessively after surgery
- Mild (5–20% factor): bleeding after surgery
- Tx: administration of appropriate coagulation factor to 40–100% of normal
- Dose of factor VIII (units) = desired rise in % factor activity $\times$ wt (kg) $\times$ 2
- Dose of plasma-derived factor IX (units) = desired rise in % factor activity $\times$ wt (kg) $\times$ 1
- Dose of recombinant factor IX (units) = desired rise in % factor activity $\times$ wt (kg) $\times$ 1.4

PREOPERATIVE ASSESSMENT

■ Perioperative correction depends on surgical procedure.

■ Low-risk examples: tooth extraction, circumcision, endo-scopy, myringotomy, port removal

■ Low-risk hemophilia A preparation: 100 mg/kg PO Amicar on morning of surgery, 100% factor VIII correction 30 minutes before surgery

■ Moderate-risk examples: T&A, synovectomy, abdominal pro-cedures

■ Moderate-risk hemophilia A preparation: 100 mg/kg PO Amicar on morning of surgery, 100% correction 30 minutes before surgery

■ High-risk examples: neurosurgery, spinal cord surgery, arthro-scopy, open heart surgery, organ transplantation

■ High-risk hemophilia A preparation: 100% correction 30 min-utes before surgery

■ Hemophilia B protocol: Amicar 100 mg/kg on morning of surgery; 100% factor IX correction 30 minutes before surgery

■ Labs: hgb, T&C

INTRAOPERATIVE MANAGEMENT

■ Careful attn to blood loss; surgical hemostasis

■ Careful positioning due to decreased joint ROM

■ Nasal intubation relatively contraindicated

■ Avoid A-line and CVP unless essential.

■ Avoid regional analgesia.

POSTOPERATIVE CONSIDERATIONS

■ Hemophilia A low risk: PO Amicar q6h × 5 d; 100% factor cor-rection 8 h after 1st dose; 50% correction 12 h after 2nd dose; 50% correction 12 h after 3rd dose; 100% correction qd × 4

■ Hemophilia A moderate risk: Amicar q6h × 5 d, 100% factor correction 8 h after 1st dose; 50% correction q12h × 6d

■ High-risk hemophilia A: 100% factor correction 8 h after 1st dose; 50% correction q12h × 15 d

- Hemophilia B: continue Amicar q6h × 5d; 100% factor IX correction 6 h after 1st dose; 50% correction 24 h after 2nd dose; length of tx depends on type of surgery
- Monitor for postop bleeding.

MITOCHONDRIAL MYOPATHY

PHILIP D. BAILEY JR., DO

BACKGROUND

- Heterogeneous group of rare disorders affecting oxidative phosphorylation; results in impaired ATP production, often presents in newborn period
- Examples: Kearns-Sayre syndrome; progressive external ophthalmoplegia; Pearson's syndrome; myoclonic epilepsy with ragged-red fibers (MERRF); mitochondrial myopathy; encephalopathy, lactic acidosis, and stroke-like episodes (MELAS)
- Ragged-red fibers (accumulation of defective mitochondria in skeletal muscle) are morphologic hallmark of these disorders.
- Clinical: single or diffuse multisystem involvement: central & peripheral nervous system, musculoskeletal, cardiac, hepatic, renal systems
- Possible: exercise intolerance, fatigue, muscle pain, progressive weakness, & cardiomyopathy
- Significant risk for adverse perioperative outcome: stroke, coma, seizures, respiratory failure, cardiac dysrhythmias, death

PREOPERATIVE ASSESSMENT

- Labs: lytes, glucose, CBC, lactate, ammonia
- IV glucose infusion to avoid metabolic crisis
- Anticipate postop admission.

INTRAOPERATIVE MANAGEMENT
- Consider A-line for glucose, ABG, and serum lactate.
- Safe anesthetic regimens are unknown: all anesthetic agents inhibit mitochondrial function.
- Avoid succinylcholine: hyperkalemia if muscle atrophy.
- Neuromuscular blockers exacerbate muscle weakness.
- Usually need controlled ventilation due to muscle weakness
- Avoid LR: baseline lactate elevated from anaerobic metabolism secondary to mitochondrial dysfunction.
- Maintain normothermia and normal pH to ensure optimal enzymatic function.
- Regional anesthesia preferred
- Sensitivity to volatile & IV anesthetic agents, including opioids

POSTOPERATIVE CONCERNS
- Decreased capacity of major organ systems
- Generalized weakness and myopathy
- Respiratory depression common after GA, opioids
- Possible cardiac dysrhythmias (e.g., heart block, pre-excitation syndrome): cardiac monitoring necessary
- Impaired hepatorenal function may prolong drug effects.
- Consider ICU for monitoring & mechanical ventilation.

MUCOPOLYSACCHARIDOSES

RONALD S. LITMAN, DO

BACKGROUND
- Lysosomal storage disorder: accumulation of acid mucopolysaccharides (heparan, keratan, & dermatan sulfates) in connective tissue of body
- Progressive skeletal & soft tissue deformities
- Early death secondary to cardiopulmonary dysfunction
- Possible cervical spine instability

- Hurler (type I): coronary artery narrowing, myocardial stiffening, valve endocardial thickening, enlarged tongue, mental retardation, joint stiffness, cervical spine immobility and/or instability, kyphoscoliosis, frequent URIs, restrictive pulmonary disease, developmental delay, hydrocephalus with increased intracranial pressure, conductive hearing loss, macrocephaly
- Hunter (type II): valvular dysfunction, coronary artery narrowing, myocardial thickening, short neck, thick tongue, upper airway obstruction, mental retardation, joint stiffness, cervical spine immobility and/or instability, hyperactivity, hydrocephalus with increased intracranial pressure, seizures
- Sanfilippo (type III): short stature, frequent URIs, developmental delay, hyperactivity, mental retardation, bulbar dysfunction with ataxia, dementia, seizures
- Morquio (type IV): valvular lesions, aortic regurgitation, short neck, midface hypoplasia, atlantoaxial instability, kyphoscoliosis
- Maroteaux-Lamy (type VI): aortic stenosis, mitral insufficiency, restrictive lung disease secondary to kyphoscoliosis, atlantoaxial instability with possible spinal cord compression, hydrocephalus with increased intracranial pressure, decreased joint mobility

PREOPERATIVE ASSESSMENT
- Focused evaluation on airway anatomy
- Std NPO times
- Normal premed if no airway abnormalities
- May require IM ketamine if uncooperative
- Antisialagogue if difficult airway
- Cervical radiographs
- Baseline neuro assessment

INTRAOPERATIVE MANAGEMENT
- Probable difficult airway after early childhood

- All sizes LMA immediately available
- No anesthetic contraindications

POSTOPERATIVE CONSIDERATIONS
- Risk of hypoxemia related to upper airway obstruction; may require prolonged intubation

---

MUSCULAR DYSTROPHY

PHILIP D. BAILEY JR., DO

BACKGROUND
- Duchenne's muscular dystrophy is most common type: 1:3,500 male births.
- Sex-linked recessive, clinically evident in males; female carriers may have subclinical abnormalities
- Cause: lack of dystrophin, component of muscle cytoskeleton, causes membrane instability & permeability, intracellular CA accumulation, cell necrosis, replacement of degenerated muscle with fibrous & adipose tissue; leads to pseudohypertrophy
- Cardiac & smooth muscle also involved
- Weakness & muscle degeneration in early childhood
- Contractures & kyphoscoliosis confine child to wheelchair by early adolescence.
- Kyphoscoliosis may cause restrictive lung disease.
- Common surgeries: muscle biopsy, contracture release, spinal fusion for scoliosis
- Death, in second or third decade, usually from CHF or pneumonia
- Severity of skeletal muscle involvement not correlated to severity of cardiac disease
- Mitral valve prolapse in up to 25%; requires SBE prophylaxis

- Becker's, Emery-Dreifuss, Limb girdle, Fascioscapulohumeral, Oculopharyngeal, and Congenital are less prevalent types; varying degrees of severity.

PREOPERATIVE ASSESSMENT
- Recent echo, CXR, PFTs, Hct
- Premedication: std; caution if hypotonic
- Fasting: std

INTRAOPERATIVE MANAGEMENT
- Delayed gastric emptying & impaired swallowing increase risk of perioperative aspiration; precautions often necessary.
- Susceptible to myocardial depressant effects of volatile agents
- Hyperkalemia from succinylcholine
- Volatile agents in DMD relatively contraindicated: rhabdomyolysis
- First indication of DMD may be cardiac arrest during general anesthesia.
- Nondepolarizing muscle relaxants may have a prolonged duration of action; use judiciously.
- Propofol for TIVA: watch myocardial fn; higher than expected doses may be required for induction.
- Use opioids with short duration of action.
- Regional anesthesia helpful

POSTOPERATIVE CONCERNS
- Recovery from paralysis may be prolonged & assoc with postop pulm complications.
- Monitor for pulm dysfunction & retained secretions.
- Decreased inspiratory, expiratory, vital & total lung capacity and decreased ability to cough predispose to postop respiratory complications.
- Delayed pulm insufficiency may occur >24 hr postop.
- Postop mechanical ventilation might be needed, especially in pts with VC <30%.

- Pulmonary toilet helpful
- Heart block may develop from fibrosis of cardiac conducting system.
- ICU admission if advanced disease

NEUROFIBROMATOSIS

RONALD S. LITMAN, DO

BACKGROUND
- Type 1: von Recklinghausen disease: café-au-lait spots; neurofibromas in skin, upper airway, and nervous system; optic gliomas; CNS tumors; kyphoscoliosis; renal artery stenosis; developmental delay
- Type 2: bilateral acoustic neuromas: hearing loss, vestibular disorientation
- Both types require frequent MRI.

PREOPERATIVE ASSESSMENT
- Focused evaluation for airway tumors
- Std NPO times
- Normal premed if no airway tumor
- May require IM ketamine if uncooperative
- BP control if renal artery stenosis

INTRAOPERATIVE MANAGEMENT
- Possible difficult ventilation with airway tumors; keep spontaneous ventilation until intubated
- No anesthetic contraindications
- TIVA if neurophysiology monitoring

POSTOPERATIVE CONSIDERATIONS
- None related to NF

OBSTRUCTIVE SLEEP APNEA

RONALD S. LITMAN, DO

BACKGROUND

- Prevalence 1–3%
- Age range: 3–6 yr
- Common in children with large tonsils, Down syndrome, craniofacial anomalies, prematurity, obesity
- Caused by combination of anatomic and neurologic abnormalities
- Most common surgical procedure is adenotonsillectomy.

PREOPERATIVE ASSESSMENT

- Child must be in optimal health to proceed with elective surgery.
- Preoperative sedation may cause upper airway obstruction; decreased dose may be warranted.
- Sleep study will give information about severity of disease based on length of apnea and SpO2 nadir.
- If long-standing or severe, cardiology consultation to rule out cardiomegaly or pulmonary hypertension
- CPAP or BiPAP therapy indicates severe disease.

INTRAOPERATIVE MANAGEMENT

- During anesthetic induction, upper airway obstruction occurs in virtually every case; manage with insertion of oral airway device.
- General anesthesia with a secured airway is preferable to moderate sedation with a natural airway for procedures involving the upper airway (e.g., endoscopy).
- Awake extubation
- May be sensitive to opioids

POSTOPERATIVE CONCERNS

- Upper airway obstruction commonly occurs, despite removal of tonsils.
- Soft nasopharyngeal airway may be required for recurrent obstruction or oxygen desaturation.
- May require relatively less opioids for postop pain control
- Postop respiratory complications related to lower age and severity of preexisting disease
- Criteria for hospital admission: age <4 yrs or when severe
- ICU admission for recurrent obstruction or oxygen desaturation

---

ONCOLOGICAL DISEASE

RONALD S. LITMAN, DO

BACKGROUND

- Leukemias: most common malignancies of childhood; lethargy, malaise, fever, pallor, ecchymoses, petechiae, bone pain, anemia, neutropenia, thrombocytopenia
- CNS tumors: most common solid tumors in children; mostly infratentorial in cerebellum & brain stem; increased ICP common: headache, nausea, emesis, lethargy, nystagmus, difficulty walking, CN deficits
- Lymphoma: Hodgkin's & non-Hodgkin's; lethargy, fevers, wt loss, anterior mediastinal mass
- Neuroblastoma: usually from adrenal medulla or thoracic paraspinal sympathetic ganglia; may have hypertension or spinal cord compression
- Wilms tumor: cancer of embryonal renal cells; painless abdominal mass, hematuria; may have IVC infiltration
- Bone tumors: Ewing's sarcoma, osteogenic sarcoma

PREOPERATIVE ASSESSMENT
- Identify side effects from chemo tx.
- Anthracyclines (Adriamycin, daunorubicin) cause cardiac toxicity: check recent echo.
- Often opioid tolerant

INTRAOPERATIVE MANAGEMENT
- Fluids: std
- Monitors: std
- No anesthetic contraindications; balanced technique
- Upper airway reflexes may be decreased.
- Meticulous detail to antisepsis, especially with indwelling venous catheters
- Careful attn to mucous membranes: mucositis from chemo tx

POSTOPERATIVE CONSIDERATIONS
- May require higher than normal opioids for analgesia

PATENT DUCTUS ARTERIOSUS

SCOTT D. MARKOWITZ, MD

BACKGROUND
- Incidence 1:2,500–5,000 births
- More common in prematures
- Usually closes spontaneously within days to wks after birth
- Persistent L to R shunting may lead to CHF & pulm hypertension if untreated.
- Surgical correction by transcatheter closure (coil or device) or surgery (thoracotomy for ligation)

PREOPERATIVE ASSESSMENT
- Hx: R/O previous recurrent laryngeal nerve injury
- BP: compare extremities
- CBC: if chronic cyanosis R/O polycythemia

■ Echo: assess residual PDA, severity of shunt, direction of flow, RV size & hypertrophy, and estimate RV pressure. R/O other CHD. Evidence of pulm htn: R to L or bidirectional shunting, RV dilation or hypertrophy, cyanosis, or RV dysfunction.
■ ECG: RVH or LVH
■ If PDA not corrected, look for pulm htn: cardio consult.

INTRAOPERATIVE MANAGEMENT
■ SBE prophylaxis indicated if PDA closed within 6 mos
■ SBE prophylaxis if residual flow or closure device implanted
■ If PDA uncorrected, be aware of PVR/SVR ratio and direction of shunting.

POSTOPERATIVE CONSIDERATIONS
■ Std analgesic regimens

POST-OPERATIVE NAUSEA AND VOMITING (PONV)

MICHAEL J. RICHARDS, BM, MRCP, FRCA

BACKGROUND
■ Prevalence higher than adults; schoolchildren up to 50%; infants 5%; preschool children 20%
■ Intractable vomiting 1–3%
■ Higher incidence in post-pubertal females
■ Increased incidence in T&A, strabismus repair, orchiopexy, herniotomy, middle ear surgery & laparotomy
■ Associated with prolonged surgical/anesthetic time & hx of motion sickness or PONV
■ Caused by stimulation of vomiting center in medulla by afferents from CTZ, vestibular apparatus, cerebellum, solitary tract nucleus, higher cortical centers & abdominal vagal nerves

PREOPERATIVE ASSESSMENT

- Identification of high-risk pts: plan antiemetic anesthetic techniques & prophylaxis
- Drug monotherapy most effective if initiated before induction of anesthesia
- Dual therapy with drugs acting on different effector sites beneficial, but not triple therapy
- Numerous classes of drugs: anti-dopamine, antihistamines, anticholinergics, anti-serotonin, steroids: none work on all stimulating receptors, none 100% effective
- Benzodiazepine premed may decrease PONV.
- Opiate premedication increases PONV.

INTRAOPERATIVE MANAGEMENT

- Induction with etomidate, ketamine, barbiturates increases PONV in adults; no data in children.
- Gastric distention during airway management by inexperienced personnel increases PONV.
- TIVA with propofol decreases PONV.
- Nitrous oxide increases PONV in certain pts.
- Opiates increase PONV; use NSAIDs or regional anesthesia when possible.
- Neostigmine reversal may increase PONV.
- Intraoperative hydration decreases PONV by decreasing need for early postop oral intake.

POSTOPERATIVE CONCERNS

- Rescue tx not as effective as prophylaxis
- Rescue tx most beneficial with different class of drug than previously used
- Pain prolongs gastric emptying & increases PONV.
- Opiates decrease pain but increase PONV.
- Variation in emetogenicity of different opiates between different pts
- Early mobilization associated with PONV

■ Consider alternative techniques; acupuncture/pressure over P6 point at wrist, perioperative suggestion, hypnosis, ginger root, alcohol sniff

---

POSTOPERATIVE APNEA

DANIEL D. RUBENS, MBBS

BACKGROUND
■ Apnea definition: resp. pause >30 sec
■ 3% of normal infants have central, obstructive, or mixed apnea associated with desaturation; 30% with concurrent URI
■ Diff dx: acidosis, hypoxia, hypoglycemia, electrolyte disturbance, anemia, sepsis, hypothermia, CNS trauma/intracranial hemorrhage
■ Factors that increase risk: lower gestational age, lower chronological age, BPD, RDS, PDA, history of apnea of prematurity, anemia, poor general health, parental smoking, pyloromyotomy (metabolic alkalosis?)

PREOPERATIVE ASSESSMENT
■ Delay elective surgery for preterm infants until beyond 44 weeks PCA.
■ Consider administration of caffeine 5–10 mg/kg in premature infants with known apnea.

INTRAOPERATIVE MANAGEMENT
■ Lower risk of postop apnea with regional procedures without sedation
■ Use of muscle relaxants and opioids increases risk.

POSTOPERATIVE CONCERNS
■ Careful monitoring of high-risk infants in PACU
■ Admit preterm infants <46 wks PCA for overnight apnea monitoring.

- Centers vary on rules; some admit up to 60 wks PCA.
- Preterm infants <44 wks PCA requiring urgent surgery: monitor at least 18 hrs; 24–36 hrs if comorbidity.
- Infants born <34 wks gestation & anemic (<10 g/dL): admit if <60 wks PCA.
- If regional alone: same rules for overnight monitoring
- <41 wks PCA for simple procedure can have apnea 12 hrs postop

---

PREMATURE INFANT

KHA M. TRAN, MD

BACKGROUND

- Prematurity = <37 wks gestation
- Low birth wt = <2,500 gm
- Very low birth wt = <1,500 gm
- Extremely low birth wt = <1,000 gm
- Maternal diabetes: congenital anomalies, macrosomia, respiratory distress syndrome, hypoglycemia
- Maternal thyroid disease: neonatal thyroid disease
- Maternal lupus (SLE): neonatal congenital heart block
- Maternal myasthenia gravis: transient neonatal myasthenia
- Maternal alcoholism: fetal alcohol syndrome
- Maternal opioid use: neonatal withdrawal syndrome
- Maternal magnesium: neonatal respiratory depression, hypotonia

PREOPERATIVE ASSESSMENT

- Current wt important for dosing drugs
- May require neonatal ventilator if severe respiratory distress syndrome
- Note current rate of dextrose infusion and trends of blood glucose to guide intraop glucose management.

■ Umbilical artery catheter should end in aorta at lumbar vertebrae level.

■ Umbilical vein catheter should end in IVC near atrium, not in liver.

■ Determine medical comorbidities:

➤ Apnea: consider regional anesthetic techniques

➤ Airway stenosis: have smaller endotracheal tubes, check for air leak around tube

➤ Bradycardia: close monitoring of heart rate, atropine premed

➤ Intraventricular hemorrhage: ensure no hydrocephalus or increased ICP (bulging fontanelles)

➤ Retinopathy of prematurity: avoid high FiO2 unless needed to avoid hypoxia

➤ Respiratory distress syndrome: appropriate ventilator settings

➤ Patent ductus arteriosus (PDA): check preductal (right hand) & postductal (left hand or toes) oxygen saturation, pulm htn & systemic hypotension may cause R to L shunt & cyanosis

➤ Indomethacin for PDA may lead to bleeding & renal dysfn.

➤ Pulm htn: avoid hypoxia, hypercarbia, acidosis, hypothermia; keep deeply anesthetized; have isoproterenol & inhaled nitric oxide available

➤ Anemia, thrombocytopenia: address cause and have blood products ready

➤ Metabolic or respiratory acidosis: address primary cause

➤ Other congenital anomalies/syndromes: specific syndromes may have implications for airway or metabolic management

INTRAOPERATIVE MANAGEMENT

■ Warm OR, forced air warming blanket, heated water mattress, active warming of breathing circuit

- Esophageal temp probe unless contraindicated
- Dextrose infusion at one-half to two-thirds preop rate. Check glucose intraop and adjust infusion as needed.
- Monitor fluid administration carefully: easy to fluid overload
- Large occiput may cause neck flexion; consider shoulder roll for intubation.
- FRC low and oxygen consumption high: preoxygenate before intubation.
- Secure endotracheal tube well: small movements cause bronchial intubation or extubation.
- Set ventilator before placing child on mechanical ventilation.
- Minimize FiO2.
- Smaller syringes result in smaller mistakes.
- Communicate with neonatal and surgical team; neonatologist can be intraoperative resource.

POSTOPERATIVE CONCERNS
- Keep infant warm during transport!
- Ensure adequate oxygen supply and means for ventilating.
- Closely monitor for postoperative apnea.

SEIZURE DISORDERS

RONALD S. LITMAN, DO

BACKGROUND
- Febrile seizures: most common type of seizure disorder in children
- Other main causes: trauma, hypoxia, infection
- Less common causes: metabolic disease, hypoglycemia, electrolyte and metabolic abnormalities, toxic ingestions, and congenital or developmental defects
- Idiopathic epilepsy: rare in children

- Partial seizure: origin limited to part of one cerebral hemisphere; motor, sensory, autonomic, or psychic phenomena
- Simple partial: consciousness not impaired
- Complex partial: consciousness impaired
- Generalized seizure: origin in both cerebral hemispheres
- Absence (petit mal): brief staring spells, pt not responsive
- Myoclonic: brief, uncoordinated twitching movements
- Tonic–clonic: initial contraction phase (may have apnea & cyanosis) followed by repetitive twitching phase
- Atonic: immobility & unresponsiveness
- Infantile spasms (West syndrome): salaam-like movements, arrest of psychomotor development, EEG pattern called hypsarrhythmia, poor prognosis
- Lennox–Gastaut: hard to control, severe mental retardation
- Carbamazepine (Tegretol): may cause leukopenia, thrombocytopenia
- Ethosuximide (Zarontin): leukopenia, aplastic anemia
- Phenobarbital: hyperactivity, sedation, nystagmus, ataxia
- Phenytoin (Dilantin): nystagmus, ataxia, lupus, gingival hyperplasia, anemia, leukopenia, polyneuropathy
- Valproic acid (Depakene, Depakote): hepatotoxicity, anemia, leukopenia, thrombocytopenia
- Gabapentin (Neurontin): dizziness, ataxia, fatigue
- Lamotrigine (Lamictal): dizziness, ataxia, double vision, Stevens–Johnson
- Levetiracetam (Keppra): somnolence, asthenia, dizziness
- Tiagabine (Gabitril): dizziness, somnolence, tremor
- Topiramate (Topamax): somnolence, fatigue, weight loss

PREOPERATIVE ASSESSMENT

- In difficult-to-control children, convert PO to IV anticonvulsants.
- In well-controlled children, anticonvulsant levels not necessary

INTRAOPERATIVE MANAGEMENT

■ Most anesthetic and analgesic agents safe

■ Exception: repeated doses of meperidine: metabolite normeperidine is proconvulsant

■ Nitrous oxide, sevoflurane, methohexital, etomidate, and all opioids anecdotally associated with seizure-like movements in healthy & epileptic pts

■ All anesthetic agents are anticonvulsants once consciousness lost.

■ Anticonvulsant use causes requirement for higher doses and shorter dosing intervals of neuromuscular blockers. Mostly for aminosteroids (vec, roc, panc).

■ Anticonvulsant use may cause some opioid resistance (1 report).

POSTOPERATIVE CONSIDERATIONS

■ Resume anticonvulsant schedule as soon as possible.

■ No known increase in seizure activity in postop period

SICKLE CELL DISEASE

PAUL G. FIRTH, MBChB

BACKGROUND

■ Congenital hemoglobinopathy, due to inheritance of hemoglobin S, a mutant variant of hemoglobin A

■ Genotypes: homozygous SS, heterozygous SC & HbS-thalassemia

■ Sickle cell trait (SCT): asymptomatic heterozygous carrier state HbAS

■ Incidence in African-American population: 0.2% for SCD, 8% for SCT

■ Clinical features: widespread vascular damage, stroke (infarction/hemorrhage), restrictive lung disease, airway hyperreactivity, hemolytic anemia, splenic enlargement/infarction,

urinary concentrating defects, renal insufficiency/failure, priapism, cholelithiasis, osteonecrosis, dactylitis, leg ulcers, shortened life expectancy
- Pain crisis: pathognomonic complication of acute pain, particularly in bones and joints, thought to be due to organ ischemia and infarction
- Acute chest syndrome: lung injury from pulmonary infection, thromboembolism or fat embolism secondary to bone marrow infarction. Dx: new lung infiltrate on CXR, chest pain, T > 38.5C, tachypnea, wheezing, cough.

PREOPERATIVE ASSESSMENT
- History: establish frequency & severity of acute complications, known precipitants, organ dysfunction
- Labs: hematocrit, creatinine, CXR if clinically indicated
- Pre-op RBC transfusion to Hgb > 10 gm/dL: may not be indicated for low-risk procedures, efficacy in moderate- or high-risk procedures controversial
- Exchange transfusion not indicated for minor- or moderate-risk procedures; possible benefit for high-risk procedures not clearly established
- Extended crossmatch for E, C, K antigen groups before transfusion

INTRAOPERATIVE MANAGEMENT
- Keep well hydrated & modify if indicated by renal pathology
- Keep well oxygenated & modify if impairment to oxygen delivery
- Keep normothermic
- Arterial tourniquet not absolutely contraindicated; use with caution
- Regional anesthetic often beneficial

POSTOPERATIVE CONCERNS
- Early mobilization, pulmonary toilet (incentive spirometry, physical therapy), effective analgesia

- Pain crisis: use pain scoring scales, opioids as needed, encourage adjuvant analgesics (NSAIDs, acetaminophen), regional analgesia, pulmonary monitoring
- Acute chest syndrome: oxygen, bronchodilators, incentive spirometry; consider broad-spectrum antibiotics
- Correction of anemia if severe hypoxia
- Mechanical ventilation for respiratory failure

SINGLE VENTRICLE PHYSIOLOGY

SCOTT D. MARKOWITZ, MD

BACKGROUND
- Hypoplastic left heart syndrome (HLHS) is most common form.
- Typically, 3 staged operations to create Fontan circulation
- Stage I (newborn period) creates modified Blalock-Taussig shunt or RV to PA shunt to provide pulmonary blood flow. Typical SpO_2 80%.
- Stage I pulmonary blood flow dependent on systemic BP.
- Stage 2 (4–6 months) removes shunt and connects SVC to pulm arteries to provide non-arterial pulmonary blood flow. Typical SpO_2 75–85%.
- Stage 3 (18 months to 4 years) adds IVC flow to pulm arteries to complete Fontan circulation and permit near-normal arterial O_2 saturation. Typical SpO_2 90–95%.
- Stages 2 and 3 pulmonary blood flow is dependent on CVP and maintaining low PVR.

PREOPERATIVE ASSESSMENT
- Ensure that SpO_2 is appropriate for pt at his/her operative stage.
- Cardiology assessment important

- Assess functional status: diminished exercise tolerance, acute weight gain or respiratory compromise.
- Echo: confirm flow in SVC, IVC and PA; show no residual coarctation of aorta; assess systolic function and AV valve function. Cath may be indicated when echo windows are poor.
- ECG: R/O arrhythmia and establish baseline
- CBC: assess level of polycythemia
- Electrolytes if on diuretic
- Keep NPO times as short as possible to ensure euvolemia.
- SBE prophylaxis

INTRAOPERATIVE MANAGEMENT
- BP lower in arm used for BT shunt
- Carefully titrated inhaled or IV induction is usually well tolerated.
- Establish IV access ASAP and appropriate fluid administration to maintain BP (stage I) and pulmonary perfusion (stages 2 and 3).
- Extreme caution when converting from spontaneous to positive-pressure ventilation in stages 2 and 3
- Ensure adequate intravascular volume; avoid high or prolonged positive airway pressures (normal pressures for normal intervals are tolerated in pts with adequate intravascular volume).
- Dopamine or epinephrine available
- Prior to extubation, optimize pulmonary function by reversing atelectasis, maintaining adequate tidal volume and pulmonary toilet.
- Recovery in ICU warranted based on pt health and response to surgery/anesthetic

POSTOPERATIVE CONSIDERATIONS
- Pain management: optimize comfort & minimize adverse effects on ventilation
- NSAIDs, acetaminophen & regional techniques

- Judicious opioid use; caution for respiratory effects
- Maintain normal intravascular volume until adequate PO intake.
- Monitor for PONV; may prevent usual medications.

TETRALOGY OF FALLOT

SCOTT D. MARKOWITZ, MD

BACKGROUND
- Incidence: approx 10% of CHD
- Consists of overriding aorta with RV outflow tract obstruction (variable degree of obstruction) + VSD
- RV hypertrophy is compensatory.
- Coexisting disease: DiGeorge syndrome (13%), pulmonary atresia (15–25%) leads to severe stenoses of branch pulmonary arteries and aorto-pulmonary collaterals in some pts; absent pulmonary valve syndrome (2%) involves dilated pulmonary arteries causing compression of bronchi. VACTERL syndrome and CHARGE association also occur with ToF.

PREOPERATIVE ASSESSMENT
- Evaluate functional status by activity level and exercise tolerance.
- ECG: arrhythmia, RV hypertrophy
- Echo: myocardial function, valvular function, rule out residual VSD
- Consider sedative premed for ages 3–9 months with history of Tet spells.
- Ensure clear liquids 2 hours prior to mask induction to maintain euvolemia.

INTRAOPERATIVE MANAGEMENT
- If pre-repair: consider cyanosis, relative polycythemia and history of hypercyanotic episode (Tet spell) to increase risk of Tet spell during induction or emergence

■ Focus on preventing hypercyanotic episode by avoiding hypovolemia, sympathetic stimulation, hypoxia and hypothermia.
■ Std monitors usually adequate
■ Induction: Ketamine for Tet spell-prone pt. Inhalation and other IV induction techniques can be safely titrated to maintain SVR and minimize PVR.
■ Adequate depth of anesthesia and normoxia may prevent a Tet spell; esmolol, phenylephrine or morphine may reverse a Tet spell.

POSTOPERATIVE CONCERNS
■ Narcotic pain management
■ Extubate when bleeding is under control and cardiorespiratory function is adequate.
■ Monitor for arrhythmias.
■ Lifelong risk may be increased for arrhythmias and sudden death.
■ Pts may require reoperation of RV outflow tract as PI worsens or conduit obstructs.
■ Physiological features after repair using transannular patch: increasing pulmonic insufficiency with RV dilation and possibly tricuspid regurgitation over time, possible atrial arrhythmias
■ Physiological features after repair using RV-PA conduit: pulmonic insufficiency and conduit obstruction after pt growth or over time leading to RV hypertrophy and dilation, possible atrial arrhythmias

---

THALASSEMIA

RONALD S. LITMAN, DO

BACKGROUND
■ Inherited decreased or defective synthesis of one or more globin chains

- Named after the affected globin chain: alpha and beta thalassemia are most common
- Unaffected globins are overproduced, cause RBC abnormalities: microcytic, hypochromic, hemolytic anemia.
- Alpha thal major: homozygous form, absence of all 4 alpha-globin chains, leads to severe fetal anemia and death (hydrops fetalis)
- Alpha thal intermedia (hemoglobin H disease): 3 alpha-globin chains absent, severe anemia, CHF, splenomegaly, jaundice, bone changes from marrow expansion due to increased RBC production
- Alpha thal trait (alpha thal minor): heterozygous form, absence of 2 alpha-globin chains, mild microcytic anemia
- Silent-carrier alpha thal: absence of 1 alpha-globin chain, hgb nl
- Beta thal major (Cooley's anemia): homozygous, absence of beta-globin chains, severe hemolytic anemia, splenomegaly, treated with chronic RBC transfusions
- Beta thal intermedia: heterozygous, moderate anemia
- Beta thal trait: absence of 1 beta chain, mild microcytic anemia
- Silent-carrier beta thal: asymptomatic
- Chronic transfusions cause iron overload.

PREOPERATIVE ASSESSMENT
- Labs: hgb, lytes, LFTs, coags
- ECG, Echo, CXR
- NPO: std
- Premedication: std, for anxiolysis
- Airway eval: look for maxillary enlargement

INTRAOPERATIVE MANAGEMENT
- Fluids: std
- Balanced anesthetic technique
- Regional if coags OK

POSTOPERATIVE CONSIDERATIONS
- None

TRANSPOSITION OF GREAT ARTERIES (D-TGA)

LUIS M. ZABALA, MD

BACKGROUND
- 5–7% of CHD; most common neonatal cyanotic lesion
- Aorta arises from anatomic RV; PA arises from anatomic LV.
- Systemic & pulmonary circ in parallel, not in series, causes cyanosis.
- Clinical presentation: hypoxemia & cyanosis shortly after birth
- Pt needs shunting at atrial, ventricular, or ductal level to survive.
- Keep ductus open with prostaglandin E1 (Alprostadil) infusion & percutaneous balloon atrial septostomy.
- Old treatments: Senning or Mustard intra-atrial baffle; 20–40% get heart failure as young adult; loss of sinus node function, tricuspid regurgitation, atrial dysrhythmias
- Current tx: arterial switch procedure: establishes normal anatomical relationship between ventricles and great arteries; long-term outcomes encouraging
- L-TGA (corrected transposition): malposition of great arteries and ventricular inversion; RA empties into anatomic LV to PA. LA empties into anatomic RV to aorta. Blood flow physiologically correct; no cyanosis but long-term tricuspid insufficiency.

PREOPERATIVE ASSESSMENT
- In children with repaired D-TGA for non-cardiac surgery, assess level of activity, cardiac reserve, & vent function.

- Preoperative sedation when appropriate: PO midazolam 0.5 mg/kg (max 10 mg) or IV midazolam 0.1 mg/kg, ketamine 0.5 mg/kg, or pentobarbital 2–4 mg/kg

INTRAOPERATIVE MANAGEMENT
- Monitors: std unless ventricular dysfunction, arrhythmias
- Balanced anesthesia technique
- Inhalational agents well tolerated

POSTOPERATIVE MANAGEMENT AND CONCERNS
- ICU for unrepaired defects, poor vent function, & after surgical repair of D-TGA
- Pts with L-TGA or surgically repaired D-TGA managed as normal following non-cardiac surgery; normal monitoring & discharge criteria normal

---

TRISOMY 21 (DOWN SYNDROME)

INGE FALK VAN ROOYEN, MBChB

BACKGROUND
- Cause: extra chromosome 21
- Incidence increases with advancing maternal age.
- Affects all races
- Males:females = 3:2
- Physical characteristics: oblique palpebral fissures, dysplastic ears, low hairline, epicanthic folds, simian crease on hand, large tongue, small mandible, short neck
- Generalized joint laxity: atlantoaxial instability, TMJ subluxation with jaw thrust
- Mild to moderate mental retardation
- Obesity
- Obstructive sleep apnea
- Hypothyroidism (6%)

- Frequent operative procedures: congenital heart disease, ear tubes, T&A, dental procedures
- 15- to 20-fold increased risk of acute megakaryocytic leukemia
- Early senile dementia

PREOPERATIVE ASSESSMENT

- Preop tests: echo, cervical spine radiographs (when clinically indicated)
- Pts may be frightened or trusting.
- Preop sedation may potentiate airway obstruction.

INTRAOPERATIVE MANAGEMENT

- Upper airway obstruction during inhalational induction common; oral airway helpful
- Subglottic stenosis: requires down-sizing endotracheal tube
- Avoid extremes of neck motion in all directions.
- Extubation best performed fully awake to prevent airway obstruction during emergence
- Judicious benzodiazepines and opioids to limit postoperative hypotonia

POSTOPERATIVE CONCERNS

- Upper airway obstruction; nasopharyngeal airway helpful
- Analgesia: ketorolac and acetaminophen to minimize opioid use
- Familiar caregiver helpful

VENTRICULAR SEPTAL DEFECT (VSD)

LUIS M. ZABALA, MD

BACKGROUND

- Most common CHD (30%), excluding PDA & bicuspid AV
- Classification based on anatomic location: perimembranous (70%), muscular (25%), supracristal (5%), inlet (5%)

- Physiologic classification based on the size of the defect, amount of shunting, & PVR/SVR
- Restrictive: small; shunt influenced by size, not SVR/PVR ratio
- Non-restrictive: large: shunt direction determined by SVR/PVR ratio
- Clinical symptoms depend on size of VSD: FTT, CHF, LV dilation & various degrees of respiratory symptoms.
- CXR: increased size of PA silhouette, LA & LV enlargement
- ECG: LA, LV hypertrophy
- Surgical closure early in childhood: excellent outcomes; survival into adulthood without sequelae
- Corrected VSD usually results in RBBB.
- Surgical correction past childhood: decreased LV function, inc PVR
- 10% with nonrestrictive VSDs develop Eisenmengers: pulm vasc obstructive disease, R to L shunt.

PREOPERATIVE ASSESSMENT
- Detailed history, meds, physical exam
- Cardiology consult may help in estimation of ventricular dysfunction & shunt-induced pulmonary htn.
- Echo: to determine size and site of the defect, direction & magnitude of shunt
- Anxiety increases L to R shunt.
- Premed: PO midazolam (0.5 mg/kg) or PO pentobarbital (4 mg/kg); caution with oversedation & hypoventilation

INTRAOPERATIVE MANAGEMENT
- Monitors: std unless long-standing L to R shunt, shunt-related pulm htn, CHF, A-fib, RV outflow obstruction
- IV & inhalation induction well tolerated
- Balance VSD shunt by controlling PVR & SVR.
- Increased SVR or decreased PVR increases L to R shunt.

- Inhalation agents, narcotics, muscle relaxants, and/or regional anesthesia usually well tolerated
- SBE prophylaxis
- Debubble all IV lines.

POSTOPERATIVE CONCERNS
- Pts with unrepaired VSD following non-cardiac surgery should be monitored closely for signs of CHF due to volume overload or atrial dysrhythmias.
- Titrate analgesics to achieve adequate pain control without depressing respiration.
- ICU admission: for pts with postop CHF, vent dysfunction, atrial or ventricular dysrhythmias, and oxygen desaturation

VON WILLEBRAND DISEASE

RONALD S. LITMAN, DO

BACKGROUND
- Most common inherited bleeding disorder; up to 1% of population
- Type 1 (~80%): decreased amounts of normal vWF
- Type 2 (~20%): decreased amounts of abnormal vWF
- Type 3 (rare): severely decreased vWF concentration & activity
- Lab: nl coags or prolonged bleeding time or PTT

PREOPERATIVE ASSESSMENT
- Hematology consult to determine response to DDAVP
- PO Amicar 100 mg/kg on morning of surgery
- If responder, 0.3 mcg/kg IV DDAVP 1 h before surgery (give over 30 min)
- DDAVP nonresponders (or types 2B or 3) get Humate-P and/or Alphanate.
- Labs: hgb, T&C when indicated

INTRAOPERATIVE MANAGEMENT

- Careful attention to bleeding; surgical hemostasis
- Nasal intubation relatively contraindicated
- Avoid A-line and CVP unless essential.
- Avoid regional analgesia, unless clearly beneficial.

POSTOPERATIVE CONSIDERATIONS

- Continue Amicar q6h × 5 d.
- 0.3 mcg/kg IV DDAVP 12 h & 24 h post-procedure (give over 30 minutes)
- Limit fluids to 2/3 maintenance for 24 h after each DDAVP dose.
- Monitor for postop bleeding.

PART TWO

Surgical
Procedures

ANTERIOR SPINAL FUSION

ORIGINALLY WRITTEN BY LUCAS TERRANOVA, MD
REVISED BY DARRYL H. BERKOWITZ, MD

COEXISTING DISEASE

- Congenital: vertebral anomalies, rib anomalies, spinal dysraphism (neural tube defects)
- Idiopathic: infantile (<3 years), juvenile (3–10 years), adolescent (>10 years)
- Neuromuscular disease: CP, polio, myopathies, syringomyelia, Friedrich's ataxia
- Associated syndromes: neurofibromatosis, Marfan's, osteogenesis imperfecta, JRA, mucopolysaccharidosis
- Neoplastic: primary or secondary disease
- Cardiac: hypertension (enlarged RV, RV Failure), mitral valve prolapse (25%)
- Pulmonary: tachypnea, wheezing, crackles – symptoms when Cobb angle >65°

PREOPERATIVE ASSESSMENT

- Determine location & degree of curvature(Cobb's angle), etiology of disease, exercise tolerance, respiratory symptoms, co-existing disease
- Neurologic: document deficits
- ECG, ECHO – assess structural disease, RV, pulmonary pressures
- Pulmonary function testing, CXR, ABG if severe
- Labs: CBC, coags, lytes, type & cross, autologous donations

PROCEDURAL CONSIDERATIONS

- Location dictates position & approach.
- Cervicothoracic (T1-T3): supine, possible removal of clavicle, manubrium & 1st rib

- Endangers great vessels, thoracic duct, nerves (brachial plexus, sympathetic chain, vagus, phrenic), esophagus, trachea, heart & lungs
- Requires one lung ventilation
- Blood loss may be rapid & large.
- Thoracic (T5–10): lateral decub, thoracotomy, DLT helpful
- Transdiaphragmatic (T10–12): approach may be retroperitoneal & transthoracic
- Lumbar: combined with posterior repair or as part of 2-stage repair
- Lateral decub retroperitoneal, or supine transperitoneal

ANESTHETIC PLAN
- Induction: dictated by patients clinical condition
- NMB: short acting agent to enable neuromonitoring
- Maintenance: TIVA, suggest propofol, remifentanil
- Monitoring: std + A-line +/- central line
- Access: large bore, peripheral
- Volume: crystalloid, albumin, PRBCs, cell saved blood, FFP, Plts, cryoprecipitate
- Special Monitoring: SSEP, MEP – communication important between tech and anesthesia to ensure optimal anesthetic management
- Some surgeons prefer wake-up test
- Emergence: analgesic plan once TIVA off: intrathecal or IV opioids
- Extubation on awakening
- Potential problems: blood loss, neurologic – from positioning or surgery, pulmonary problems related to surgical correction, pain

PAIN MANAGEMENT
- Systemic: intraop opioid infusion; titrate down at end
- Regional: intrathecal morphine, 0.005 mg/kg, after induction or intraop by surgeon under direct vision

- Intraop monitoring precludes local anesthesia in regional.

PACU/POSTOPERATIVE CONSIDERATIONS
- Analgesia: PCA or opioid infusion
- Pt should be comfortable & alert for neuro assessment.
- Neuro assessment precludes regional with local anesthesia.
- Intrathecal morphine lasts 12–18 h.

APPENDECTOMY

RICHARD ROWE, MD, MPH

CO-EXISTING DISEASES
- Vomiting, dehydration, ileus, possible peritonitis

PREOPERATIVE ASSESSMENT
- Studies: CBC, lytes
- Premed: titrate IV midazolam
- NPO: N/A–full stomach
- Correct dehydration
- Antibiotics: depends on signs of sepsis/peritonitis

PROCEDURAL CONSIDERATIONS
- Monitors: std; consider CVP, Foley if sepsis or A-line if CV instability
- IV fluids: LR: deficit + maint + 3rd space (7–10 mL/kg/h); add glucose if hypoglycemic
- Risks: hypoglycemia if NPO > 24 h, regurgitation & aspiration at induction
- Decompress stomach with OG tube after intubation

ANESTHETIC PLAN
- Offer spinal to older children.
- GA: RSI: propofol or pentothal, NMB with sux or roc.
- Maintenance: air, O_2, volatile agent; avoid N_2O
- Awaken & extubate in OR

PAIN MANAGEMENT
- Systemic: titrate opioid of choice
- Local anesthesia by surgeon
- Avoid central neuraxial block if pt septic

PACU/POSTOPERATIVE CONSIDERATIONS
- Analgesia: PCA morphine

ARTERIAL SWITCH PROCEDURE FOR TRANSPOSITION OF THE GREAT ARTERIES

MICHAEL P. EATON, MD

CO-EXISTING DISEASES
- VSD, patent foramen ovale, PDA
- CHF, cyanosis
- Aberrant coronaries

PREOPERATIVE ASSESSMENT
- Performed in infancy or as 2nd stage after PA banding or BT shunt
- Contraindicated if fixed high PVR, LV deconditioning, or possibly LV outflow obstruction
- Studies: hct, lytes if on diuretic, baseline SpO_2
- Cardiac cath or echo to define anatomy, LV function, ?VSD or LV outflow obstruction, coronary anatomy
- Preop balloon atrial septostomy PRN & PGE1 to increase mixing & SPO_2
- Premed: none
- NPO: std

PROCEDURAL CONSIDERATIONS
- Supine, typically moved away from head of table after intubation & lines
- Sternotomy

- Fluids: LR/NS ± colloid. Consider dextrose-containing fluid if failure to thrive, sick neonate, or on D10/TPN.
- Blood available
- Small infants need low dead-space access to central circulation for pressors & heparin.
- Sufficient venous access for sudden hemorrhage
- Have available: epinephrine, phenylephrine, calcium, heparin
- Monitors: std + A-line, CVP, Foley, core temp, TEE important for assessing repair
- Risks: death, bleeding, stroke, LV failure
- CPB: neonates may require more heparin (400 units/kg)
- Substantial hemodilution with CPB, may need platelets/FFP
- For circ arrest, topical cooling for head, consider pharmacologic neuroprotection (STP)

ANESTHETIC PLAN
- Goals: maintain HR, contractility & preload
- Keep ductus open with PGE1: 0.1 mcg/kg/min
- Avoid increases in PVR relative to SVR
- Induction: high-dose IV fentanyl 50-100 mcg/kg + pancuronium
- If no IV, IM ketamine/atropine ± sux
- Maintenance: may add low-dose volatile agent for BP control
- Emergence: intubated to ICU
- Adjuvant tx: hyperventilation, 100% FIO_2 unless VSD large with high pulmonary blood flow
- Pacemaker available
- Temp >36 & adequate inotropy before weaning CPB
- Follow ABGs

PAIN MANAGEMENT
- Systemic: residual opioid adequate, consider fentanyl infusion through ICU transfer

PACU/POSTOPERATIVE CONSIDERATIONS
- Coronary artery kinking can cause ischemia.
- Bleeding
- Ensure proper transfer of care to ICU physician.

ATRIAL SEPTAL DEFECT REPAIR

MICHAEL P. EATON, MD

CO-EXISTING DISEASES
- Other cardiac defects, esp VSD (AV canal) & anomalous pulmonary venous return (sinus venosus ASD)
- May have significant RV dysfunction
- Frequent pulmonary infections

PREOPERATIVE ASSESSMENT
- Studies: hct, lytes if on diuretic, baseline SpO_2
- Echo, or less commonly cardiac cath to define anatomy, shunt, ventricular fn
- Premed: midazolam, omit if neonate or cyanotic
- NPO: std

PROCEDURAL CONSIDERATIONS
- Supine: move away from head of table after intubation & lines
- Sternotomy
- IV fluids: LR/NS ± colloid
- Blood available
- Small infants need small dead-space access to central circulation for pressors, heparin, etc.
- Sufficient venous access for sudden hemorrhage
- Have available: epi, phenylephrine, calcium, heparin
- Monitors: std + A-line, CVP, Foley, core temp, TEE

- Risks: death, bleeding, stroke, RV failure
- CPB: neonates may require more heparin (400 U/kg)
- Small infants substantially hemodiluted with CPB may need platelets/FFP.

ANESTHETIC PLAN
- Mask sevoflurane in O_2 or 50% N_2O induction for healthy younger pts
- If IV present: pentothal or propofol
- If significant RV dysfunction, high-dose opioid, etomidate or ketamine
- NMB for intubation; pancuronium will decrease bradycardia with high-dose opioid
- Maintenance: inhalational + low- to moderate-dose fentanyl/sufentanil consistent with postop plans
- Avoid N_2O around CPB & with pulmonary hypertension
- Emergence: healthy pts with uneventful intraop course may be extubated in OR
- Small infants and pts with pulmonary hypertension and/or RV dysfunction may be left intubated in ICU.
- Adjuvant tx: pacemaker available
- Temp >36 and adequate inotropy before weaning CPB

PAIN MANAGEMENT
- Systemic: low- to moderate-dose fentanyl/sufentanil
- Consider fent infusion to ICU for pts needing postop ventilation
  - ➤ Consider single-shot caudal morphine at end of case (0.05 mg/kg).

PACU/POSTOPERATIVE CONSIDERATIONS
- If extubated in OR, consider risks of transport with unprotected airway.
- Ensure proper transfer of care to ICU physician.

AWAKE CRANIOTOMY FOR SEIZURES

RONALD S. LITMAN, DO

CO-EXISTING DISEASES
- Seizure disorder unresponsive to conventional therapy
- Varied etiologies of seizures

PREOPERATIVE ASSESSMENT
- Studies: hct, T&S
- Don't need anticonvulsant levels
- Document baseline neuro status.
- Assess potential for upper airway obstruction during conscious sedation.
- Premed: avoid midazolam, alternative: Benadryl 1 mg/kg PO or IV
- NPO: std

PROCEDURAL CONSIDERATIONS
- Pt needs to respond and vocalize during craniotomy while surgeon determines location of seizure focus to be removed by cortical electrodes.
- Light sedation required
- Local anesthesia to scalp & periosteum: pt can be more deeply sedated before actual mapping for seizure focus
- Brain tissue insensible to pain
- Pt should be as awake as possible during mapping.
- Position: usually lat decub
- IV fluids: LR; 3rd space losses 3–6 mL/kg/h
- Monitors: std; capnograph on nasal cannula
- Risks: hypoxia from upper airway obstruction, anxiety & lack of cooperation may lead to induction of GA; exacerbation of seizures; nausea/vomiting

ANESTHETIC PLAN

- Mild to moderate sedation achieved with use of low-dose opioids + propofol infusion: titrate to keep pt conscious & comfortable
- Adjuvant tx: surgeon may request mannitol, furosemide and/or dexamethasone

PAIN MANAGEMENT

- Local anesthesia by surgeon + opioid during procedure

PACU/POSTOPERATIVE CONSIDERATIONS

- Analgesia: opioids rarely needed
- Possible increased seizures or new neuro deficits

BIDIRECTIONAL GLENN OR HEMI-FONTAN PROCEDURE

SUANNE DAVES, MD

CO-EXISTING DISEASES

- Procedures physiologically similar: provide systemic venous to PA blood flow by creation of a superior cavopulmonary anastomosis (SVC to PA connection)
- Both interim steps for surgical treatment of single ventricle physiology (final step is completion Fontan)
- In single ventricle physiology, creation of SVC to PA anastomosis removes volume load of ventricle & allows remodeling & optimization of diastolic dimensions needed for Fontan
- Contraindicated in neonatal period when PVR & pulmonary vasoreactivity may preclude adequate passive systemic venous to PA flow

PREOPERATIVE ASSESSMENT

- May see varying degrees of cyanosis with polycythemia
- Determine underlying defect & cardiac reserve (ECHO)
- Likely to have "pre-Glenn" cath data – Raised PVR, poor function, AV valve regurgitation of stenosis, atrial arrhythmias,

restrictive atrial defects may preclude adequate passive pulmonary blood flow.

PROCEDURAL CONSIDERATIONS

- Supine: median sternotomy
- Pts may have had previous sternotomies for palliation of excessive pulmonary blood flow (PA banding), inadequate pulmonary blood flow (BT shunt), or systemic ventricular outflow obstruction (aortic arch reconstruction.
- Consider antifibrinolytics.
- Determination of transpulmonary gradient possible with IJ and common atrial pressure measurements
- Bidirectional Glenn may not require cross-clamp.

ANESTHETIC PLAN

- Premed: if >1 yr, PO midazolam 0.5–1 mg/kg; max 20 mg
- Mask induction may not be well tolerated in hypoplastic left ventricle pts.
- Maintenance: volatile agents determined by myocardial reserve
- Weaning from CPB: in contrast to completion Fontan, increases in PVR are usually well tolerated & result only in increased cyanosis. CO maintained since IVC blood continues to return to common atrium (physiologic left atrium).
- Pulmonary blood flow dependent on adequate intravascular volume & transpulmonary gradient

PAIN MANAGEMENT

- Epidural or IV opioids
- NSAIDs vs. acetaminophen with normal renal function and normal coagulation parameters (usually POD 1)

PACU/POSTOPERATIVE CONSIDERATIONS

- Elevation of PA pressures, ventricular dysfunction or stenosis at anastomosis will decrease pulmonary blood flow.
- Hypo- vs. hypercarbia to enhance pulmonary blood flow controversial

■ Return to spontaneous ventilation may improve pulmonary blood flow.

BONE MARROW ASPIRATION & BIOPSY

PAUL TRIPI, MD

CO-EXISTING DISEASES
■ Blood disorder or malignancy
■ Anemia, thrombocytopenia, immunosuppression, fever & chronic illness
■ Chemotherapy complications: Adriamycin (doxorubicin): cardiotoxicity; vincristine: peripheral neuropathy; bleomycin: pulmonary fibrosis

PREOPERATIVE ASSESSMENT
■ Studies: CBC
■ Premed: midazolam (omit if using propofol)
■ NPO: std

PROCEDURAL CONSIDERATIONS
■ Position: usually prone for BM bx; prone or lateral for LP
■ Often performed out of OR
■ Usually <15 minutes
■ IV fluids: any
■ Monitors: std
■ Risks: when out of OR, appropriate resources (O_2, suction, airway equipment, emergency drugs) immed available
■ Pts with immunosuppression or neutropenia will need isolation room & sterile technique; swab IV ports with alcohol.

ANESTHETIC PLAN
■ Depending on pt's age & level of anxiety, conscious or deep sedation with combination of opioids or benzodiazepines, or deep sedation with propofol

- GA with sevoflurane or IV/IM ketamine is acceptable alternative.
- Conscious or deep sedation: titrate IV midazolam & fentanyl to desired level of responsiveness & resp stability
- Unconscious sedation: propofol bolus ($\pm$ infusion) either alone or added to above agents
- ETT sometimes necessary for difficult airway or full stomach
- Adjuvant tx: antiemetic if prone to PONV

PAIN MANAGEMENT
- Systemic: titrate opioid
- Regional: subQ local anesthetic

PACU/POSTOPERATIVE CONSIDERATIONS
- Pts recover quickly; may bypass PACU if alert, oxygenating & ventilating without difficulty, & minimal nausea/vomiting/pain
- Analgesia usually unnecessary

BRANCHIAL CLEFT CYST EXCISION

ORIGINALLY WRITTEN BY RICHARD VAX, MD,
AND DOLORES B. NJOKU, MD
REVISED BY DOLORES B. NJOKU, MD

CO-EXISTING DISEASES
- Branchio-oto-renal syndrome: renal insufficiency, mandibular & palate defects
- DiGeorge syndrome: abnormal thymus & parathyroid (hypocalcemia), cardiac defects & choanal atresia
- Goldenhar's syndrome: facial asymmetry, mandibular hypoplasia, difficult airway
- Treacher-Collins: mandibular hypoplasia, difficult airway

PREOPERATIVE ASSESSMENT
- Studies: if lesion large, CT or MRI: to eval airway anatomy
- Premed: if >8 months, PO midazolam 0.5 mg/kg; max 15 mg
- NPO: standard for age

PROCEDURAL CONSIDERATIONS
- Supine; head often turned to side
- IV fluids: LR or NS $\pm$ dextrose (2.5 or 5%) (in infants)
- Monitors: std
- Risks: airway edema, additional facial nerve injury
- Blood loss minimal

ANESTHETIC PLAN
- Mask or IV induction of choice
  - ➤ Maintenance: volatile agent & N_2O
  - ➤ Avoid NMB if monitoring facial nerve
  - ➤ Awaken & extubate in OR

PAIN MANAGEMENT
- Titrate opioid of choice to alertness, RR and HR
- Local anesthetic in incision by surgeon
- Rectal acetaminophen (30–40 mg/kg)

PACU/POSTOPERATIVE CONSIDERATIONS
- Airway swelling, additional facial nerve injury
- Usually acetaminophen 10–15 mg/kg PO q4h or 30–40 mg/kg (initial rectal dose) followed after 6 h by 20 mg/kg (PR) q6h is sufficient for pain.
- Rarely IV fentanyl 0.5–1 mcg/kg (or other opioid of choice)

BURN DEBRIDEMENT

SAM SHARAR, MD

CO-EXISTING DISEASES
- Inhalation injury with airway obstruction, V/Q mismatch, CO intoxication, difficult intubation

- Hypovolemia with burns >20% body surface area; fluid loss at burn sites & generalized capillary leak
- Painful wounds/prolonged opioid use leads to tolerance.

PREOPERATIVE ASSESSMENT
- Studies: hct; ABG if inhalation injury
- Premed: titrate IV midazolam and/or opioid
- NPO: std; continue enteral tube feedings intraop in critically ill pts due to high metabolic needs

PROCEDURAL CONSIDERATIONS
- Donor harvest supine (thigh); prone (back/buttock); intraop repositioning for burn excision or grafting
- IV fluids: 3rd space & sensible (including hemorrhage) fluid losses large & unpredictable, dependent on burn size/depth; indirect volume indicators (BP, HR, urine output, serial hcts) helpful; replace with LR & RBC blood products; be wary of large crystalloid volumes injected subcutaneously by surgeons to facilitate donor skin harvest: may lead to volume overload
- Monitors: std, Foley; if multiple burned extremities may need facial pulse oximeter, "needle" EKG electrodes & A-line for BP/serial hematocrits; CVP rarely indicated, unless no peripheral IV access
- Risks: hypothermia (poor skin integrity, exposure & fluid replacement): increase room temp & use fluid warmers; loss of airway or vasc access during repositioning: carefully secure ETT & IV lines

ANESTHETIC PLAN
- Difficult airway or no IV access: mask induction with sevo +/− N_2O
- Easy airway with IV access: IV induction
- FOB-assisted intubation may be required if facial burns/edema.

- NMBs for intubation if easy airway: large burns result in non-depolarizing NMBs; avoid sux: hyperkalemia risk with burns >48 h
- ETT usually required
- Maintenance: balanced technique: O_2, N_2O, volatile agent
- Generous titration of opioids: anticipate significant postop pain with opioid tolerance
- Awaken & extubate in OR

PAIN MANAGEMENT
- Systemic: fentanyl or morphine or hydromorphone
- Regional: caudal or lumbar epidural, extremity block for lower extremity burns

PACU/POSTOPERATIVE CONSIDERATIONS
- Analgesia: systemic opioids
- Anticipate opioid tolerance.
- Orthotic devices on extremities, head/neck may limit IV/airway access.
- Sedation/immobility may be requested to protect fragile skin grafts.

CARDIAC CATHETERIZATION

ORIGINALLY WRITTEN BY PEDRO VANZILLOTA, MD
REVISED BY DARRYL H. BERKOWITZ, MD

CO-EXISTING DISEASES
- Structural heart disease
- Vascular disease (e.g. aortic coarct, anomalous venous drainage, pulmonary vasc disease)
- Cardiac transplant

PREOPERATIVE ASSESSMENT
- Detailed history & exam

- Labs: Hgb important in cyanotic disease (correct if low)
- ABG (if pt critically ill)
- PT, PTT, Plts
- Lytes: important if pt on diuretics, low systemic output, or nephrotoxic drugs (transplant pts/antibiotics).
- ECHO: delineate anatomy, ventricular function, fluid collections
- CXR: vascular congestion, consolidation, cardiac shadow size, effusions, ETT position, line placements
- Head ultrasound: gross abnormalities & ventricular hemorrhage in neonates, if planned anticoagulation
- Abdominal ultrasound: assess organ abnormalities
- Premed: midazolam, pentobarbital, meperidine all OK, topical local anesthetic for access sites
- Avoid sedative premed if direct myocardial depression or vent depression dangerous

PROCEDURAL CONSIDERATIONS

- Indications: diagnosis of CHD, define anatomy, hemodynamic measurements (Qp:Qs), arterial & venous saturations, assess myocardial fn, angiography, endomyocardial biopsies.
- Interventional: valvotomy (balloon dilation across stenotic valve), angioplasty (on native vessels – e.g., coarct post-surgery or surgical conduits), endovascular stents, closure of shunts, electrophysiological studies & radiofrequency ablation

ANESTHETIC PLAN

- Induction: may include ketamine, fentanyl, midazolam
- If pulm htn, avoid depressed myocardial fn at induction; acute changes in SVR or PVR dangerous.
- Maintenance: balanced technique – muscle relaxant, volatile anesthetic

- FiO2 depends on clinical situation (most caths performed at room air).
- Fluids: little more than maintenance except with acute blood loss or if high filling pressures needed (e.g., TOF)
- Ventilation: spontaneous or controlled; keep EtCO2 near-normal for accurate hemodynamic calcs
- Monitoring: std + A-line from cath site
- Position: arms may be above head – monitor stretch on brachial plexus
- Adequate padding to legs & pressure points
- Urinary catheter for long cases
- Blood available for all cases
- Emergence: reversal, antiemetic, minimal straining to minimize bleeding from puncture sites
- Complications: hypothermia, cardiac deterioration, arrhythmias, bleeding at puncture site, vessel damage, cardiac tamponade, air or fragment embolism, contrast allergy, acute hemodynamic changes – valvular incompetence, acute changes in pulmonary or systemic flow

PAIN MANAGEMENT
- IV fentanyl, local for insertion site

POSTOPERATIVE CONSIDERATIONS
- Recovery depends on disease, pre- & post-procedure cardiac fn, interventions.
- ICU: pts with intraop hemodynamic or rhythm disturbance, ongoing Qp:Qs imbalance with hypoxemia or poor systemic output
- Pulm htn pts: high post-cath morbidity & mortality in 1st 24 hrs
- Supine for up to 6 h if groin puncture
- Analgesia: acetaminophen, fentanyl

CERVICAL NODE BIOPSY/EXCISION

RONALD S. LITMAN, DO

CO-EXISTING DISEASES

- Often presenting sign of lymphoma or leukemia; suspect mediastinal mass & ask about symptoms: cough or dyspnea when supine raises suspicion
- If leukemia: anemia, thrombocytopenia, & neutropenia
- May have been on chemotx if known malignancy
- Most common dx: infection or reactive lymph node; suspect TB if pt in population at risk or has chest symptoms

PREOPERATIVE ASSESSMENT

- Studies: CBC if suspect malignancy
- CT of chest or neck if suspect lymphoma: R/O mediastinal mass or tracheal compression by neck mass
- If known mediastinal mass with tracheal compression, avoid GA unless absolutely indicated for tissue dx before tx (see chapter on anterior mediastinal mass)
- Premed: PO midazolam 0.5 mg/kg; max 10 mg; avoid if signs of upper airway obstruction preop
- NPO: std

PROCEDURAL CONSIDERATIONS

- Supine with head turned away from lesion
- Usually limited access to airway during procedure
- IV fluids: LR; 3rd space loss minimal
- Monitors: std

ANESTHETIC PLAN

- Inhalation induction with sevoflurane or IV induction with agent of choice
- NMB of choice may be used to facilitate intubation

- ETT required
- LMA possible but not advised because airway not easily accessible
- Maintenance: balanced technique with N_2O, O_2, & volatile agent
- Awaken & extubate in OR

PAIN MANAGEMENT
- Systemic: opioids usually not necessary but small doses of fentanyl or morphine OK
- Regional: local infiltration by surgeon

PACU/POSTOPERATIVE CONSIDERATIONS
- Analgesia: PO acetaminophen or ibuprofen
- Low chance of bleeding into neck

CHOLEDOCHAL CYST EXCISION

RONALD S. LITMAN, DO

CO-EXISTING DISEASES
- Cyst obstructs bile drainage: results in jaundice-direct hyperbilirubinemia
- Varying degrees of severity of jaundice depending on duration of obstruction before dx
- May have liver damage by the time of dx

PREOPERATIVE ASSESSMENT
- Studies: hct, T&C, coags, LFTs
- Premed: if >1 yr, PO midazolam 0.5 mg/kg; max 10 mg
- NPO: std

PROCEDURAL CONSIDERATIONS
- Supine; RUQ incision
- IV fluids: LR; 3rd space loss 10–12 mL/kg/h
- May require FFP if liver damage caused abnormal coags

- IV fluids warmed
- Usually little blood loss but potential for intraop bleeding, esp if abnormal coags
- Monitors: std
- Risks: hypothermia: increase temp in OR, forced warm air blanket underneath & around child & HME in breathing circuit
- Hypovolemia: from unanticipated bleeding or 3rd space loss from bowel exposure

ANESTHETIC PLAN

- Inhalation induction with sevoflurane or IV induction with agent of choice
- NMB may be used to facilitate intubation.
- ETT required
  - Maintenance: balanced technique with O_2, air, & volatile agent
- Titrate opioids if no regional.
- Avoid N_2O to prevent bowel distention.
- Awaken & extubate in OR.

PAIN MANAGEMENT

- Systemic: titrate fentanyl to hemodynamics but limit use to avoid vent depression at end of procedure
- Morphine, alfentanil, sufentanil, & remi acceptable alternatives
- Regional: intraop epidural anesthesia by insertion of catheter via caudal canal after induction of anesthesia & placement of ETT
- Local anesthetic choices: 3% 2-chloroprocaine, 0.1–0.2% ropivacaine, or 0.25% bupivacaine

PACU/POSTOPERATIVE CONSIDERATIONS

- Analgesia best accomplished by continuation of epidural meds

- Choices: 2% 2-chloroprocaine, or 0.0625–0.125% bupivacaine
- Avoid epidural narcotics in pts <1 yr
- Systemic: IV morphine 0.05 mg/kg prn

CIRCUMCISION

PASQUALE DE NEGRI, MD

CO-EXISTING DISEASES
- None

PREOPERATIVE ASSESSMENT
- Studies: none
- Premed: if >1 yr, PO midazolam 0.5 mg/kg; max 15 mg
- NPO: std

PROCEDURAL CONSIDERATIONS
- Supine
- IV fluids: LR at maintenance
- Minimal blood or 3rd space loss
- Monitors: std

ANESTHETIC PLAN
- Standard inhalation induction with sevoflurane or IV induction with propofol or thiopental
- NMB not usually required
- LMA or mask: spont ventilation
- Maintenance: balanced technique: $N_2O + O_2$ + volatile agent
- Avoid opioids if regional used
- Awaken and remove LMA in OR.

PAIN MANAGEMENT
- Systemic: titrate fentanyl or alfentanil if no regional
- Regional: penile or caudal block
- Methods for penile block: bilat dorsal penile nerve blocks; ring block; or subpubic space block

- Use 0.25% plain levobupivacaine or bupivacaine or 0.2% ropivacaine 2–4 mL total
- Types of topical creams:
  - ➤ Tetracaine (AMETOP) & EMLA
  - ➤ Both helpful but not as good as regional

PACU/POSTOPERATIVE CONSIDERATIONS
- Pain: PR acetaminophen 40 mg/kg, then 20 mg/kg q6h

CLEFT LIP REPAIR

LUCINDA EVERETT, MD

CO-EXISTING DISEASES
- Feeding difficulties may lead to poor growth & anemia.
- Difficult airway or cardiac defects in various syndromes
- Usually performed at 2–3 mo; some centers advocate repair earlier in infancy
- Older children may return for cosmetic repairs of lip & nasal tip.

PREOPERATIVE ASSESSMENT
- Studies: none
- Consider hct in infants with failure to thrive or prematurity.
- Premed: usually none; midazolam for older or agitated infants
- NPO: std

PROCEDURAL CONSIDERATIONS
- Supine; pt's head near end of OR table turned 90°
- IV fluids: deficit + maintenance; minimal 3rd space or blood loss
- Monitors: std
- Hyperthermia possible if using warming blanket
- Risks: depend on assoc diseases or airway issues
- Statistically, risk is slightly higher in children <1 yr.

■ Surgeon may inject local anesthetic w/epinephrine.

ANESTHETIC PLAN
■ Inhalation induction; NMB may be used to facilitate intubation
■ Place oral RAE tube in midline; secure with waterproof tape; confirm bilat breath sounds in surgical position.
■ Maintenance: volatile agent + N_2O; spontaneous or controlled ventilation; cautious amts of opioid: fentanyl 0.5–2 mcg/kg or morphine 0.025–0.05 mg/kg
■ Emergence: extubate awake; adequate analgesia helps minimize crying & subsequent bleeding or swelling at suture line

PAIN MANAGEMENT
■ Systemic: titrate small amts of opioid; PR acetaminophen 30–40 mg/kg
■ Regional: local by surgeon or infraorbital nerve blocks

PACU/POSTOPERATIVE CONSIDERATIONS
■ Soft arm restraints often used to keep infant from disrupting suture lines.
■ Analgesia: nerve block/local; acetaminophen with cautious use of opioid

CLEFT PALATE REPAIR

LUCINDA EVERETT, MD

CO-EXISTING DISEASES
■ Nasopharyngeal reflux, chronic aspiration with possible lung disease, poor nutritional status due to feeding difficulties
■ Associated with syndromes that may involve difficult intubation (Pierre-Robin), cardiac or renal lesions & hypotonia
■ Elective repair usually performed by 12–18 mo of age

■ Procedures in later childhood include velopharyngeal flap or repair of bony palatal defects with bone graft.

PREOPERATIVE ASSESSMENT
■ Studies: none
■ Premed: midazolam if needed; give PR if difficult oral intake
■ NPO: std

PROCEDURAL CONSIDERATIONS
■ Supine; pt's head extended & near end of OR table turned 90°
■ Surgeon injects local anesthetic w/epi.
■ IV fluids: deficit + blood loss
■ Blood loss usually minimal, but occasionally can be significant & not readily apparent.
■ Monitors: std
■ Hyperthermia possible if using warming blanket
■ Risks: difficult airway with induction in certain pts; may have obstruction on emergence & postop

ANESTHETIC PLAN
■ Usually inhalation induction; equipment available for difficult airway in syndromic pts
■ Intubation not difficult in most pts, but cleft is visually distracting & laryngoscope can catch in cleft
■ NMB may be used to facilitate intubation; spontaneous respiration preferred if difficult airway anticipated.
■ Oral RAE tube; confirm bilat breath sounds with head extended in surgical position
■ Maintenance: balanced technique; spontaneous or controlled ventilation
■ Throat pack usually used
■ Watch for airway obstruction with placement of mouth gag.
■ Emergence: suction under direct vision or along tongue to avoid disrupting suture line

- Extubate awake; anticipate possibility of airway obstruction due to anatomic changes + blood & edema.
- Surgeon may place tongue suture in all or selected pts to rapidly open airway if needed postop.
- Adjuvant tx: consider suctioning stomach, particularly if throat pack is saturated; antiemetic; dexamethasone

PAIN MANAGEMENT
- Cautious doses of opioid
- Ketorolac may be contraindicated because of bleeding issues.
- Regional: local by surgeon

PACU/POSTOPERATIVE CONSIDERATIONS
- Analgesia: acetaminophen; cautious use of opioid
- Airway issues & positioning
- Arm restraints often used

CLOACAL EXTROPHY REPAIR

PASQUALE DE NEGRI, MD

CO-EXISTING DISEASES
- Abdominal wall defect with intestine exposed; bladder split & completely exposed
- External genitalia malformed
- Pelvic kidneys; unilateral renal agenesis; polycystic kidney; ureteral duplication
- Vertebral anomalies
- GI anomalies (omphalocele, imperforate anus)
- Spinal defects (myelomeningocele)
- Lower extremity deformities

PREOPERATIVE ASSESSMENT
- Studies: hct, lytes, T&C
- Premed: usually none

■ NPO: empty stomach; NG or OG tube placed at birth

PROCEDURAL CONSIDERATIONS

■ Surgery on 1st DOL to repair omphalocele & close bladder & usually colostomy
■ Subsequent surgeries are staged reconstructions of external genitalia.
■ Supine
■ IV fluids: warmed LR, 5% albumin;
■ 3rd space losses >15 mL/kg/h
■ Blood loss & transfusion common
■ Monitors: std + A-line + CVP
■ Risks: bleeding, hypothermia: use forced warm air blanket underneath & around pt & HME in circuit

ANESTHETIC PLAN

■ Inhalation induction with sevoflurane or IV induction with agent of choice; ketamine if unstable hemodynamics
■ NMB to facilitate intubation: prefer cisatracurium since no liver metabolism
■ ETT required
■ Maintenance: balanced technique: O_2, air, volatile agent
■ Decision when to awaken & extubate will depend on fluid status, temp & length of surgery.

PAIN MANAGEMENT

■ Systemic: titrate opioid of choice to hemodynamics
■ Regional: caudal epidural catheter for intraop & postop use
■ Local anesthetic choices: 0.2% ropivacaine, 0.25% levobupivacaine or bupivacaine or 3% chloroprocaine

PACU/POSTOPERATIVE CONSIDERATIONS

■ Hypothermia, hypovolemia, restoration of autonomous ventilation & analgesia

- Epidural analgesia: 0.0625–0.125% levobupivacaine (max 0.25 mg/kg/h)
- Systemic: IV morphine 0.05–0.1 mg/kg prn

CLUBFOOT REPAIR

LAKSHMI VAS, MD

CO-EXISTING DISEASES
- Additional congenital anomalies: 12%
- Muscular dystrophy: possible MH association
- Cerebral palsy

PREOPERATIVE ASSESSMENT
- Studies: none
- Premed: PO/PR/nasal midazolam
- NPO: std

PROCEDURAL CONSIDERATIONS
- Position: semi-lateral, may require change of position for circumferential correction
- Tourniquet usually used; don't exceed 75 min at inflation to 150 mmHg
- More than 1 inflation needed for major correction
- IV fluids: warmed LR or equivalent
- 3rd space loss: 6–8 mL/kg/h
- IV in the upper extremity
- Blood loss: minimal
- Temp loss: minimal if covered
- HME in breathing circuit

ANESTHETIC PLAN
- Inhalation induction: O_2, N_2O, sevoflurane
- IV: pentothal 4–6 mg/kg or propofol 3–4 mg/kg or ketamine 1.5–2 mg/kg preceded by 0.25 mg/kg midazolam

- Maintenance: if short procedure: spontaneous ventilation with LMA & $N_2 O/O_2$ & isoflurane
- Longer: intubation, controlled ventilation, NMB, or Proseal LMA with spontaneous ventilation with concomitant regional anesthesia
- Awaken & extubate in OR.

PAIN MANAGEMENT

- Systemic: titrate opioid of choice
- Regional: single-shot or continuous caudal/lumbar epidural
- Single-shot or continuous sciatic & femoral block for unilateral anesthesia
- Local anesthetic choices: 0.5% bupivacaine, max 2.5 mg/kg; 2% ropivacaine, max 2.5 mg/kg; 3% 2-chloroprocaine, max 11 mg/kg; 2% lidocaine, max 5 mg/kg

PACU/POSTOPERATIVE CONSIDERATIONS

- Good analgesia important for extremely painful foot surgery
- Epidural/sciatic block infusion: 0.0625–0.125% bupivacaine, 0.2–0.4 mg/kg/h; 0.1% ropivacaine, 0.2 mg/kg/h
- Epidural narcotics relatively contraindicated <6 mo age
- Systemic: fentanyl preferred if regional not present

CNS TUMOR EXCISION

ORIGINALLY WRITTEN BY SANDRA KAUFMAN, MD
REVISED BY DOLORES B. NJOKU, MD

CO-EXISTING DISEASES

- Hydrocephalus: increased ICP with supra- & infratentorial tumors, Cushing's triad (late)
- Cranial nerve impairment: loss or compromise of gag reflex could result in aspiration pneumonia
- May require modified RSI

- Hypoventilation could worsen increased ICP; abnormal CO_2 response curve may be exacerbated by mask induction
  - Cerebral salt-wasting syndromes (very rare): may need to correct sodium to pt's baseline
- Peripheral neuropathy: document with abbreviated neurological exam before induction; maintain neutral positioning of extremities & head

PREOPERATIVE ASSESSMENT
- Studies: MRI or CT, hct, coagulation profile, others as per preop hx
- Premed: none or minimal if inc ICP
- NPO: full stomach if presentation urgent or compromised gag reflex

PROCEDURAL CONSIDERATIONS
- Position depends on tumor location.
- IV fluids: NS
- Monitors: std + A-line, SSEP
- Central venous line for tx of VAE or if peripheral access poor
- Risks: blood loss, VAE, neurological deficits, herniation, cerebral edema, airway edema

ANESTHETIC PLAN
- IV induction preferable
- Mask induction OK if CNS symptoms absent
- Maintenance: balanced technique: volatile agent, O_2, N_2O & NMB
- Awaken & extubate in OR if neuro assessment and airway OK
- Adjuvant tx: dexamethasone for tumor-induced vasogenic edema

PAIN MANAGEMENT
- Intraop: opioid of choice, at induction 5–10 micrograms/kg for a 4-hour procedure

■ Titrate opioid of choice to alertness, RR and HR after emergence from anesthesia
■ May use acetaminophen 10–15 mg/kg PO q4h or 30–40 mg/kg (initial rectal dose) followed after 6 h by 20 mg/kg (PR) q6h

PACU/POSTOPERATIVE CONSIDERATIONS
■ ICU admission, frequent neuro assessment

COARCTATION OF THE AORTA REPAIR

SCOTT WALKER, MD

CO-EXISTING DISEASES
■ Aortic hypoplasia, bicuspid AV, AS, TOGV
■ Preductal coarc assoc w/ CHF
■ CHF worsened by PDA, VSD & mitral disease
■ Ductal & postductal coarc less symptomatic

PREOPERATIVE ASSESSMENT
■ Studies: echo and/or cath, CXR, ABG
■ Premed: none for young infants; if >1 yr, PO midazolam 0.5 mg/kg; max 15 mg
■ NPO: std

PROCEDURAL CONSIDERATIONS
■ Position: R lat decub
■ IV fluids: avoid overhydration, esp with CHF or pts w/ VSD
■ Blood immed available in OR
■ Monitors: R radial A-line, distal A-line or NIBP; avoid L arm (L SCA may be sacrificed)
■ SSEP if indicated
■ Consider cerebral and/or somatic oximetry.
■ Cool to 35°C (spinal cord protection)
■ Risks: spinal cord ischemia; worse in minor coarcs (poor collaterals)

- Inc risk if distal MAP <45 mmHg, clamp time >20 min, or hyperthermia
- Adjust cross-clamp or place shunt if distal MAP <45 mmHg or somatic oximetry low
- Phrenic or recurrent laryngeal n injury
- Avoid hyperventilation: dec CBF

ANESTHETIC PLAN
- Induction: if preductal & unstable: fentanyl + ketamine + NMB
- If stable or no IV access: sevo OK
- If ductal or postductal: sevo; STP or propofol if IV present
- Maintenance: remifentanil + volatile agent
- Atropine if HR decreases with ductal manipulation
- If keeping intubated postop: fentanyl 30–50 mcg/kg + low-dose volatile agent or benzo
- Awaken & extubate in OR if: good analgesia, CXR OK & normothermia

PAIN MANAGEMENT
- Systemic: remi 0.2–1.0 mcg/kg/min if planning to extubate; if keeping intubated, liberal titration of any opioid
- Regional: local infiltration, intercostal block or retropleural catheter with continuous infusion of lidocaine
- Caudal morphine 0.05 mg/kg
- Some avoid neuraxial analgesia to prevent confounding dx of neuro changes from spinal cord ischemia.

PACU/POSTOPERATIVE CONSIDERATIONS
- Hypertension: tx w/ nitroprusside ± esmolol
- Analgesia: morphine, meperidine, or hydromorphone prn or PCA in appropriate pts
- IV ketorolac 0.3 mg/kg q6h prn

COLONOSCOPY

SURESH THOMAS, MD

CO-EXISTING DISEASES
- Hematochezia
- Occult GI bleeding
- Unexplained chronic diarrhea
- Surveillance for malignancy, ulcerative colitis, Gardner's syndrome
- Inflammatory bowel disease
- Intestinal polyposis

PREOPERATIVE ASSESSMENT
- Studies: none, unless indicated by hx
- Premed: midazolam PO or IV prn
- SBE prophylaxis in at-risk pts
- EMLA cream
- NPO: std

PROCEDURAL CONSIDERATIONS
- Position: lateral decubitus/supine
- IV fluids: LR at maintenance after replacing deficits
- Monitors: std
- Risks: abdominal distention, hypoxemia, hypotension, bacteremia, cardiac arrhythmias (electrolyte imbalance & hypovolemia from bowel prep), vasovagal reflex, rarely hemorrhage & bowel perforation

ANESTHETIC PLAN
- Induction: consider RSI in severe GERD
- If no aspiration risk, mask or IV induction of choice
- Airway mgt options include ETT, LMA, nasal cannula, face mask with or without oral or nasal airway.

- Maintenance: O_2, air & volatile agent $\pm$ opioid
- In older children, deep sedation: propofol 75–200 mcg/kg/min $\pm$ fentanyl 1–2 mcg/kg
- Emergence: if intubated, extubate when awake

PAIN MANAGEMENT
- Systemic: short-acting opioids preferred
- Regional: none

PACU/POSTOPERATIVE CONSIDERATIONS
- Analgesia: PO acetaminophen 10–15 mg/kg prn q4h
- IV morphine 0.05 mg/kg q5–10 min prn
- PONV: consider IV ondansetron 0.1 mg/kg (max 4 mg)

CONGENITAL CYSTIC ADENOMATOID MALFORMATION (CCAM) EXCISION

MIKE MAZUREK, MD

CO-EXISTING DISEASES
- CCAMs are cystic, solid, or mixed intrapulmonary masses that communicate with the normal tracheobronchial tree.
- Newborns born with CCAM display early respiratory distress when lesions are large.
- Usually involves only a single lobe
- Likely assoc congenital heart disease
- May displace mediastinum to contralateral side
- Differential dx includes congenital lobar emphysema, bronchogenic cyst, tension pneumothorax, sequestered lobe, & pneumonia with pneumatocele formation.
- Recurrent infections & pulmonary abscesses

PREOPERATIVE ASSESSMENT
- CXR & CT scan to evaluate extent of mediastinal shift, airway impingement, & infection

- Studies: H/H, T&C
- Premed: if >1 yr, PO midazolam
- NPO: std

PROCEDURAL CONSIDERATIONS

- Lobectomy via thoracotomy
- Prevent further enlargement of cyst by avoiding PPV with awake intubation or inhalation induction.
- Use low inflating pressures if assisted ventilation necessary.
- Avoid N_2O.
- If cyst enlargement occludes airway or causes cardiovascular compromise, needle aspiration or emergent thoracotomy may be life-saving.
- If cyst fluid-filled or infected, selective bronchial blocking may protect unaffected lung.
- Monitors: std + A-line

ANESTHETIC PLAN

- Inhalational induction: avoid high PIP
- Consider bronchial blocker.
- Maintenance: opioids + volatile agent + NMB

PAIN MANAGEMENT

- Systemic: titrate IV fentanyl
- Regional: intercostal nerve block; caudal catheter threaded to thoracic level using local anesthetics and/or opioids

PACU/POSTOPERATIVE CONSIDERATIONS

- Hypoxemia, hypoventilation

CONGENITAL DIAPHRAGMATIC HERNIA REPAIR (CDH)

MIKE MAZUREK, MD

CO-EXISTING DISEASES

- Pulmonary hypoplasia (ipsilateral and contralateral lungs)

- Persistent pulmonary hypertension
- Associated congenital heart disease common

PREOPERATIVE ASSESSMENT
- Studies: H/H, T&C
- Medical mgmt until respiratory & cardiovascular systems stabilized
- Tx includes high-frequency ventilation, ECMO, inhaled NO, & surfactant replacement

PROCEDURAL CONSIDERATIONS
- Supine
- IV fluids: LR + prn glucose
- Monitors: std + A-line; consider central line for intraop & postop use
- Risks: pneumothorax on contralateral side, hypoxemia, hypercarbia, hypothermia
- Abdominal or thoracoabdominal approach
- Large defects require artificial diaphragm for closure
- Abdominal silo used to stretch abdominal cavity when necessary
- Repair possible while pt on ECMO or high-frequency ventilation

ANESTHETIC PLAN
- Most pts come to OR intubated
- Induction: opioids, volatile agent, NMB
- Pre- & post-ductal SpO_2 will help diagnose R-to-L shunting.
- R radial A-line for monitoring preductal gases
- Do not attempt to expand hypoplastic lung. High peak inspiratory pressures may cause pneumothorax on nonoperative side.

PAIN MANAGEMENT

- Systemic: titrate fentanyl
- Regional: consider caudal catheter threaded to thoracic level if early extubation considered

PACU/POSTOPERATIVE CONSIDERATIONS

- Pulmonary hypertension, hypoxemia, persistent PDA
- Postop analgesia: systemic opioids if intubated; regional also possible

---

CONGENITAL LOBAR EMPHYSEMA

LAKSHMI VAS, MD

CO-EXISTING DISEASES

- 10–37% incidence of VSD or PDA
- Bronchomalacia
- Redundant bronchial mucosa
- Bronchial stenosis
- Abnormal vessels or lymph nodes may cause extrinsic pressure & emphysema.
- Respiratory distress
- Emphysematous lobe compresses normal lung, raises intrathoracic pressure, reduces venous return & cardiac output.

PREOPERATIVE ASSESSMENT

- Studies: echo if suspect CHD
- CXR to assess mediastinal shift
- Premed: none if <6 mo
- NPO: std

PROCEDURAL CONSIDERATIONS

- Position: lateral decub

- Lobectomy or pneumonectomy
- IV fluids: warmed LR or equivalent
- 3rd space loss 7–10 mL/kg/h
- IV in nondependent upper extremity
- Blood loss usually minimal
- Monitors: std
- Risks: overdistention of emphysema with positive-pressure ventilation
- Hypothermia: increase OR temp
- Warming blanket underneath & around pt during surgery
- HME in breathing circuit

ANESTHETIC PLAN

- Preoxygenation
- Inhalation induction with O_2, sevoflurane
- Titrate IV ketamine 1.5–2 mg/kg also OK
- Attempt spontaneous ventilation until chest open
- Avoid N_2O.
- If bronchoscopy: spray larynx with lidocaine
- Spontaneous ventilation through ventilating bronchoscope
- After bronchoscopy, trachea intubated for thoracotomy
- Endobronchial intubation has been described to avoid over-inflation of emphysematous lung.
- Once chest open, use NMBs.
- Maintenance: O_2, air, volatile agent
- Awaken & extubate in OR.

PAIN MANAGEMENT

- Systemic: titrate fentanyl or other opioid
- Regional: epidural catheter via lumbar or caudal approach; can thread up to T4–6 area
  - ➤ Consider tunneling caudal catheter to avoid soiling from urine & feces. Continuous paravertebral block is another option for unilateral anesthesia.

- Local anesthetic choices: 0.25% bupivacaine, max 2.5 mg/kg; 3% 2-chloroprocaine, max 11 mg/kg; 2% lidocaine, max 5 mg/kg

PACU/POSTOPERATIVE CONSIDERATIONS
- Respiratory physiotherapy
- Good analgesia important for adequate ventilation
- Epidural medication infusion: 0.0625–0.125% bupivacaine at 0.2–0.4 mg/kg/h
- Epidural opioids relatively contraindicated <6 mo
- Systemic: fentanyl preferred if no regional

CRANIOSYNOSTOSIS REPAIR

ORIGINALLY WRITTEN BY LES GARSON, MD
REVISED BY DARRYL BERKOWITZ, MD

CO-EXISTING DISEASES
- Syndromes (eg, Apert, Crouzon, Treacher Collins, etc): assoc with difficult airway
- Neurological: Sagittal suture – ICP normal, >1 suture: may have elevated ICP, mental retardation, impaired brain growth
- Respiratory: usually normal but if associated with midface hypoplasia, choanal atresia may have chronic hypoxia & pulmonary hypertension, RVH, cor pulmonale
- Cardiac: evaluate for associated anomalies, pulmonary hypertension

PREOPERATIVE ASSESSMENT
- Studies: H/H, T&C, coags
- Premed: anxiolytic if >8 mos
- NPO: std
- Discuss transfusion with parents
- Blood available (<7 days old or if older washed to avoid hyperkalemia)

- Continue all cardiac, seizure medication but discuss with surgeon any anticoagulant therapies
- Drugs ready: antibiotics, calcium, resuscitative meds & infusions

PROCEDURAL CONSIDERATIONS
- Prone or supine, OR table turned 90°
- IV fluids: LR, 12–15 mL/kg/h due to large surface area exposed & large 3rd space loss
- Potential for large & rapid blood loss: need 2 IVs usually in feet (saphenous) & ready availability of PRBCs or whole blood
- Monitors: std, Foley, A-line, consider precordial Doppler
- CVP optional: used for access & potential evacuation of air embolus
  - Risks: major blood loss, ICP elevations, hypothermia, hyperkalemia, hypocalcemia, air embolism, facial and airway swelling
- If >1 blood volume transfused, consider FFP + platelets.
- BP & character of A-line tracing can indicate volume status.
- Hypothermia: use warmed IV fluids, forced warm air blanket around infant, increase OR temp
- Air embolism potentially significant
- Cerebral edema: may need hyperventilation & diuresis

ANESTHETIC PLAN
- Induction: maintain spont ventilation until positive-pressure ventilation ensured
- Careful attention to securing ETT & protecting pressure points
- Maintenance: balanced technique: air, O_2, volatile agent, opioids
- Avoid N_2O.
- Volume replacement: Hb >10, consider starting with 10 mL/kg PRBC
- Hb <10, consider 20 mL/kg PRBC on incision.

- Use balanced solution – NS may induce hyperchloremic acidosis.
- Remember K load and hypocalcemia from citrate with ongoing transfusions.
- Important to keep up with losses
- Ongoing metabolic acidosis indicates hypovolemia.
- Consider cell salvage, antifibrinolytics.
- If ICP elevated, consider hyperventilation, mannitol, furosemide.
- Awaken & extubate in OR if airway mgmt uneventful.
- Adjuvant tx: surgeon may request mannitol

PAIN MANAGEMENT
- Systemic: titrate fentanyl during case; avoid toward closure
- Regional: local anesthetic to incision by surgeon

PACU/POSTOPERATIVE CONSIDERATIONS
- Recovery in ICU: transfer on full monitoring with emergency airway equipment, emergency drugs, volume available, suction on bed
- Analgesia: morphine 0.05 mg/kg prn
- Serial H/H for 1st 24 h: oozing continues postop
- Airway obstruction from facial edema
- Monitor continued drainage of blood, coags & PLTs

CRANIOTOMY FOR HEAD TRAUMA

MONICA S. VAVILALA, MD

CO-EXISTING DISEASES
- Cervical spine injury
- SCIWORA (spinal cord injury without radiologic abnormalities)
- Facial & airway trauma

PREOPERATIVE ASSESSMENT
- Studies: head CT, hct, INR, fibrinogen, PTT, plts, T&C
- Premed: none

PROCEDURAL CONSIDERATIONS
- Supine with head up, lateral, park bench, or prone depending on injury site
- IV fluids: 2 catheters; warmed LR, Plasmalyte, or NS
- Monitors: std + Foley
- A-line after induction
- Risks: excess hyperventilation, hypothermia, hypotension, increased ICP, hemorrhage, cerebral edema, herniation, death

ANESTHETIC PLAN
- IV induction (avoid ketamine)
- RSI: sux or roc
- Mild hyperventilation before tracheal intubation if signs of herniation
- In-line neck stabilization
- Maintenance: balanced technique: NMBs, air, O_2, volatile agent
- Avoid N_2O: may inc ICP before dura open & after dura closed
- Opioids OK during induction; avoid at end of case
- May need to keep intubated until post-surgery CT done
- Adjuvant tx: phenytoin, mannitol, furosemide, $PaCO_2$ 30–35 mmHg
- Keep SBP/MAP/CPP age-appropriate.
- Transfuse when hct in low 20s
- Postop ICP monitoring
- Pentothal, propofol, etomidate, or lidocaine to decrease ICP

PAIN MANAGEMENT
- Systemic: minimal
- Regional: none

PACU/POSTOPERATIVE CONSIDERATIONS
- For transport to head CT: propofol or midazolam + NMB
- SIADH, diabetes insipidus, inc ICP
- Analgesia: minimal; opioids usually not required

CRYOTHERAPY FOR RETINOPATHY OF PREMATURITY (ROP)

DEBASHISH BHATTACHARYA, MD

CO-EXISTING DISEASES
- ROP: vasoproliferative disorder of retina in premature infants & leading cause of blindness
- Associated problems:
- Airway–subglottic stenosis (smaller ETT)
- Lungs: bronchopulmonary dysplasia (may require inc PIP)
- Metabolic: hypoglycemia, hypocalcemia
- Cryotherapy performed in first few months of life to avascular part of retina
- Approximate duration: 30 min

PREOPERATIVE ASSESSMENT
- Studies: consider hct, glucose, lytes for sick preemie
- Premed: none
- NPO: std

PROCEDURAL CONSIDERATIONS
- Supine
- IV fluids: D5 0.2 NaCl or LR for maintenance
- Monitors: std

- Risks: airway problems: bronchospasm, pulmonary edema, endobronchial intubation
- Hypothermia possible; use warming measures: increase temp in OR, warming mattress
- Keep infant well covered.

ANESTHETIC PLAN
- Inhalation or IV induction for pts with IV
- Mask anesthesia, LMA or intubation acceptable
- Short-acting NMBs may facilitate intubation.
- Maintenance: O_2/air or O_2/N_2O + inhalation agent
- Limit intraoperative narcotic use (eg, fentanyl 1 mcg/kg) to minimize risk of postop apnea.

PAIN MANAGEMENT
- Procedure associated with minimal pain
- Analgesia: PO acetaminophen 15 mg/kg q4h or PO ibuprofen 5–10 mg/kg q6h

PACU/POSTOPERATIVE CONSIDERATIONS
- Infants of post-conceptual age <50 wk are at risk of postop apnea for 12–24 h: admit for observation.
- Most infants successfully extubated at completion of procedure

---

CT SCANS

RONALD S. LITMAN, DO

CO-EXISTING DISEASES
- Can have any coexisting disease
- CT commonly performed for oncologic and pulmonary disease

PREOPERATIVE ASSESSMENT

- Studies: none
- Premed: usually none but if necessary and >1 yr, PO midazolam 0.5 mg/kg, max 10 mg
- Consider parent present during induction
- NPO: std; radiologists often require oral contrast shortly before scan

PROCEDURAL CONSIDERATIONS

- Usually supine but can be prone
- Need lead shield over reproductive organs
- IV fluids: any
- Monitors: std
- Some scans require arms over head.

ANESTHETIC PLAN

- Inhaled or IV induction
- May need RSI if emergency or recent oral contrast
- Alternative: secure ETT and then administer oral contrast via orogastric tube
- Anesthesiologist stays inside (with lead coat) or outside scanner.
- Airway mgmt depends on clinical situation & anesthesiologist pref: ETT, LMA, oral/nasal airway, or nasal cannula
- Maintenance: TIVA or inhalational
- TIVA (propofol 200 mcg/kg/min) if anesthesia machine unavailable

PAIN MANAGEMENT

- None required

PACU/POSTOPERATIVE CONSIDERATIONS

- Proactively determine plan for emergence either at scanner or PACU.

CYSTIC HYGROMA (LYMPHATIC MALFORMATION) EXCISION

ORIGINALLY WRITTEN BY YVON BRYAN, MD
REVISED BY RONALD S. LITMAN, DO

CO-EXISTING DISEASES

- Potential difficult airway if large; extrinsic compression on trachea
- Associated lymphangiomas of tongue cause difficulty with mask ventilation & LMA/ETT placement.

PREOPERATIVE ASSESSMENT

- Studies: none; H/H if large lesion & suspect blood loss
- MRI or CT to delineate anatomy
- Premed: none if <1 yr; PO/PR midazolam for older children; if difficult airway & planning awake intubation: atropine, ketamine, & midazolam carefully titrated
- NPO: std

PROCEDURAL CONSIDERATIONS

- Supine with head turned to side or extended for exposure
- IV fluids: LR or NS
- Add dextrose if <6 mo.
- Monitors: std; consider A-line if expecting large blood loss or need ABGs
- Risks: loss of airway on induction or extubation during head movement; blood loss, hypothermia

ANESTHETIC PLAN

- Induction: depends on risk of difficult intubation
- If lesion small & normal airway, inhalation or IV induction OK

- If lesion large with suspected difficult intubation or ventilation, keep pt spontaneously breathing; perform inhalation induction & place LMA or ETT with pt ventilating spontaneously.
- If unable to visualize vocal cords place LMA then ultrathin fiberoptic bronchoscope for ETT placement.
- Safe alternative: awake fiberoptic intubation after topicalization of airway & light sedation
- Last resort: awake tracheostomy under local, but may be difficult if mass is midline or large
- Maintenance: balanced technique; titrate fentanyl
- If small lesion, awaken & extubate in OR; leave intubated if lesion large with potential for airway edema

PAIN MANAGEMENT
- Systemic: titrate opioids
- Regional: none

PACU/POSTOPERATIVE CONSIDERATIONS
- Airway edema
- Residual bleeding
- Analgesia: titrate morphine 0.05 mg/kg prn

DENTAL EXTRACTIONS & REHABILITATION

RONALD S. LITMAN, DO

CO-EXISTING DISEASES
- Many pts have comorbidities (eg, cancer, developmental delay, mental retardation & seizures).

PREOPERATIVE ASSESSMENT
- Studies: none
- Premed: PO midazolam 0.5 mg; max 10 mg
- NPO: std

PROCEDURAL CONSIDERATIONS
- Supine
- OR table may be turned to side.
- Limited access to airway during procedure
- IV fluids: LR; 3rd space loss minimal
- Monitors: std
- Risks: nasal bleeding from intubation, undetected disconnect or obstruction of breathing circuit under drapes; obstructed $ETCO_2$ tubing under drapes; hyperthermia if warming measures used
- Soften nasal tube by storing in warm water, or use lubricated red rubber catheter as introducer.
- Adjuvant tx: 0.05% oxymetazoline spray to each nasal passage to lessen bleeding with nasal intubation; avoid phenylephrine spray

ANESTHETIC PLAN
- Inhalation/IV induction of choice
- NMB helps facilitate nasal intubation.
- Nasal intubation OK in all ages
- Use nasal RAE & secure to forehead with taped head wrap.
- Use same size nasal ETT as oral.
- Magill forceps usually necessary to pass nasal ETT through glottis
- Maintenance: balanced technique: N_2O & inhalational agent
- Awaken & extubate in OR.

PAIN MANAGEMENT
- Intraop: fentanyl 1–2 mcg/kg or morphine 0.05 mg/kg
- PR acetaminophen 40 mg/kg
- Local anesthesia by dentist

PACU/POSTOPERATIVE CONSIDERATIONS
- Nasal bleeding
- Analgesia for gum soreness: acetaminophen PO 10–15 mg/kg and/or PO ibuprofen 10 mg/kg

DORSAL RHIZOTOMY

ORIGINALLY WRITTEN BY JUAN PABLO GRIMALDOS, MD
REVISED BY RONALD S. LITMAN, DO

CO-EXISTING DISEASES

- Spastic cerebral palsy: GE reflux, hydrocephalus, cognitive impairment, seizures, bronchopulmonary dysplasia, reactive airway disease
- Multiple sclerosis
- Chronic pain conditions
- Post-spinal cord injury

PREOPERATIVE ASSESSMENT

- Studies: none
- Premed: if >10 mo, PO midazolam 0.5 mg/kg; max 10 mg
- NPO: std

PROCEDURAL CONSIDERATIONS

- Prone position unless unilateral cervical rhizotomy (done in lateral decubitus position)
- May need intraop X-ray
- IV fluids: warmed LR or NS
- 3rd space loss 7–10 mL/kg/h
- Minimal to moderate blood loss
- Monitors: std + Foley
- EMG + SSEP monitoring possible
- Risk of hypothermia, nerve injury or pressure ulcers

ANESTHETIC PLAN

- Inhalation induction with sevoflurane
- Rapid or modified rapid sequence if severe GE reflux or IV induction with any agent
- Short- to intermediate-acting NMB to facilitate intubation
- Intubation required

- Maintenance: O_2/N_2O or air, inhalational agents & opioids; avoid NMBs to facilitate EMG monitoring intraop
- TIVA also acceptable alternative
- Surgeon may ask for Valsalva maneuver to check for dural leak.
- Awaken & extubate in OR.

PAIN MANAGEMENT
- Systemic: fentanyl titrated at end of case, then start at 1–2 mcg/kg/h or morphine 10–20 mcg/kg/h
- Regional: consider epidural catheter after intubation or surgically placed
- Local anesthetic choice: 0.1% bupivacaine (max 0.2 mg/kg/h in infants <6 mo or 0.4 mg/kg/h in older pts), or 1.5% lidocaine
- If children >1 yr, opioids in epidural: fentanyl 1 mcg/kg/h

PACU/POSTOPERATIVE CONSIDERATIONS
- CSF leak
- Epidural bleeding
- Severe pain
- Urinary/bowel dysfunction
- Neurological impairment
- Meningitis

ENDOSCOPY – EGD (ESOPHAGOGASTRODUODENOSCOPY)

SURESH THOMAS, MD

CO-EXISTING DISEASES
- Esophageal stricture
- GERD
- Hematemesis/melena
- Foreign body ingestion
- Recurrent abdominal pain, nausea, vomiting, diarrhea, weight loss

- Ulcers
- Portal vein hypertension

PREOPERATIVE ASSESSMENT

- Studies: none, unless indicated by hx
- Premed: SC or IV midazolam prn
- Consider H_2 antagonists and/or metoclopramide
- EMLA cream
- SBE prophylaxis in pts at risk
- NPO: std

PROCEDURAL CONSIDERATIONS

- Position: lateral decub/supine
- IV fluids: LR at maintenance after replacement of deficits
- Monitors: std
- Risks: hypoxemia, aspiration, ETT migration, gastric distention, rarely bleeding & perforation

ANESTHETIC PLAN

- Induction: consider RSI in severe GERD
- Succinylcholine may trigger MH in susceptible pts, cause cardiac arrest in myopathic pts; hence it is best avoided in children when possible.
- If no aspiration risk, mask or IV induction of choice
- Maintenance: balanced technique: volatile agent, O2, air ± opioid
- In older children, consider deep sedation with propofol 75–200 mcg/kg/min ± fentanyl or remifentanil.
- Awaken & extubate awake.

PAIN MANAGEMENT

- Systemic: titrate short-acting opioid to effect

PACU/POSTOPERATIVE CONSIDERATIONS

- Vomiting: consider IV ondansetron 0.1 mg/kg (max 4 mg)

- Analgesia: PO acetaminophen or IV morphine 0.05 mg/kg q5–10 min prn

---

EPIGLOTTITIS

CHERYL K. GOODEN, MD, FAAP

CO-EXISTING DISEASES

- Acute fulminant bacterial infection usually caused by *H. influenzae* type b
- Includes all supraglottic structures, with potential for complete airway obstruction
- Dyspnea, dysphagia, dysphonia, drooling (4 Ds), severe sore throat
- Fever can exceed 40 C
- Pt agitated & toxic-appearing
- Symptoms progress rapidly.

PREOPERATIVE ASSESSMENT

- Studies: none
- Premed: none
- Pts with epiglottitis should receive supplementary O_2, be kept calm (parent present), sitting position, constant observation
- Transport to OR ASAP
- Pt must be accompanied to OR by anesthesiologist, ENT, nurse & all necessary airway & resuscitation equipment.

PROCEDURAL CONSIDERATIONS

- OR prepared with various-sized oral styletted ETTs: age-appropriate & smaller
- IV fluids: any
- Monitors: std
- Risks: life-threatening complete airway obstruction
- Instruments for emergency tracheotomy & bronchoscopy on standby

ANESTHETIC PLAN

- Sitting on parent's lap for induction
- Inhalation induction with O_2 & slow increase in concentration of sevoflurane
- Pt must be deeply anesthetized before laryngoscopy.
- Avoid paralysis for intubation: spontaneous ventilation helps identify glottic opening if swollen or inflamed.
- After oral intubation & pt well oxygenated & anesthetized, oral tube can be removed & replaced with nasal ETT.
- Nasal ETT better tolerated if prolonged intubation
- Switch of ETT from oral to nasal is left to the discretion of the anesthesiologist.

PAIN MANAGEMENT

- Not usually required

PACU/POSTOPERATIVE CONSIDERATIONS

- ICU admission
- Sedation to tolerate ETT
- Pt intubated for 24–48 h until airway swelling resolves & leak detected
- Blood and throat cultures
- Antibiotic therapy

ESOPHAGEAL DILATATION

CATHY BACHMAN, MD

CO-EXISTING DISEASES

- Esophageal strictures usually secondary to underlying pathology
- Repaired TEF
- Esophageal scarring: caustic ingestion; foreign body; other physical or chemical injury
- If caustic ingestion, possible upper airway scarring

■ Esophagus proximal to obstruction may be dilated & contain pooled secretions or food.

PREOPERATIVE ASSESSMENT
■ No labs if child well
■ Consider H/H & lytes if dehydrated or cachectic
■ Child may be very apprehensive if has undergone multiple anesthetics for dilatation.
■ Multiple premedication options: PO/PR midazolam 0.5 mg/kg; IV midazolam or opioid – titrate to effect
■ NPO: std
■ Esophagus may remain "full" proximal to stricture, despite adequate fasting.
■ SBE prophylaxis if indicated

PROCEDURAL CONSIDERATIONS
■ Supine or lateral decub
■ Table may be turned 90°
■ Sometimes indeterminate length

ANESTHETIC PLAN
■ Modified RSI with cricoid pressure & intubation
■ IV fluids: LR, deficit & maintenance
■ Maintenance: ensure immobility by deep anesthesia or paralysis
■ Monitor adequacy of ventilation during procedure; trachea at risk for compression
■ Awake extubation in OR

PAIN MANAGEMENT
■ Discomfort usually mild
■ Systemic: small doses of opioid or NSAID or acetaminophen if PO allowed

PACU/POSTOPERATIVE CONSIDERATIONS

- Observe for signs of esophageal perforation, including severe pain, tachycardia, fever, pneumothorax, or mediastinal air on X-ray.
- Analgesia: postop discomfort usually not severe
- If pain severe, consider significant tissue damage, including esophageal tear or perforation & potential for development of mediastinitis.

ESOPHAGEAL FOREIGN BODY REMOVAL

RICHARD ROWE, MD, MPH

CO-EXISTING DISEASES

- Usually none

PREOPERATIVE ASSESSMENT

- Pts usually have full stomach.
- Proceed only if life-threatening.
- Otherwise follow std NPO guidelines to lessen risk of aspiration.
- Investigate size, shape, & position of object and effect on child.
- Obtain X-ray just before case to confirm location of object.
- Premed: IV midazolam
- NPO: N/A-full stomach if foreign body obstructs esoph & pool of saliva develops

PROCEDURAL CONSIDERATIONS

- Monitors: std
- IV fluids: LR: maint + deficit
- Risks: aspiration of fluid proximal to foreign body

ANESTHETIC PLAN

- GA induction: consider RSI with propofol + sux or roc if emergent or if accumulation of saliva proximal to foreign body
- ETT required
- Omit cricoid pressure if in region of foreign body.
- Maintenance: O_2, N_2O, isoflurane
- Awaken & extubate in OR

PAIN MANAGEMENT

- Systemic: titrate low-dose fentanyl

PACU/POSTOPERATIVE CONSIDERATIONS

- Analgesia: may require low-dose opioid

EXPLORATORY LAPAROTOMY FOR ABDOMINAL TRAUMA

MONICA S. VAVILALA, MD

CO-EXISTING DISEASES

- Splenic & liver injuries
- Chest injuries: 15% mortality
- Pelvic and LE fractures: suspect if lower abdominal injury
- Always consider head injury.

PREOPERATIVE ASSESSMENT

- Studies: abdominal CT or DPL, CXR, hct, T&C
- Premed: none unless agitated

PROCEDURAL CONSIDERATIONS

- Supine
- IV fluids: 2 large-bore IV catheters; warmed LR, Plasmalyte or NS
- If no IVs, insert intraosseous line in long bone.
  - ➤ 3rd space loss >10 mL/kg/h
- Blood loss can be significant.
- Monitors: std + Foley, A-line if unstable

- Central venous cannulation if major abdominal vascular injury or major liver/splenic injury
- Hypothermia possible; use warming measures: increase temp in OR, forced warm air blanket, HME in breathing circuit
- Risks: hemorrhagic shock, death

ANESTHETIC PLAN

- IV induction: etomidate or ketamine if in shock
- RSI: use sux or roc + volume expansion
- Maintenance: volatile agent (SEVO or ISF) + opioids
- Orotracheal intubation
- NG tube if no basilar skull fracture; else OG tube
- NMBs
- Extubate in OR if awake preop & stable hemodynamics during case.
- Anticipate transfusion early.
- Cell saver if no bowel injury

PAIN MANAGEMENT

- Systemic: opioids
- Avoid regional if coags unknown, hemodynamic instability, unknown coexisting injuries.

PACU/POSTOPERATIVE CONSIDERATIONS

- Nausea & vomiting: consider prophylactic ondansetron
- Postop analgesia: opioids
- PCA for appropriate pts

FETAL SURGERY

JEFFREY GALINKIN, MD

CO-EXISTING DISEASES

- Maternal:
  - Gastric: aspiration, reflux

- ➤ Pulm: dec FRC, inc O_2 consumption
- ➤ CV: hypotension: dec preload
- ➤ CNS: sedation & weakness; dec MAC, inc sensitivity to NMB
- Fetal:
  - ➤ CV: dec Starling curve; dec baroreflex, dec blood volume, inc vagal tone
  - ➤ CNS: dec MAC, receives less agent than mother
  - ➤ Skin: inc evaporation, inc heat loss, inc bruising
  - ➤ Coags: inc bleeding
- Uteroplacental:
  - ➤ Premature labor: inc risk from uterine manipulation
  - ➤ Relaxation: flaccid uterus required
  - ➤ Perfusion: inc uterine blood flow from high-dose inhalation anesthetics
  - ➤ Hemorrhage: bleeding due to uterine relaxation

PREOPERATIVE ASSESSMENT
- Studies: maternal ultrasound with fetal echo, maternal T&C, maternal CBC, glucose, UA
- Premed: metoclopramide 10 mg IV, sodium bicitrate 30 mL PO
- NPO: std

PROCEDURAL CONSIDERATIONS
- Supine & L uterine displacement
- IV fluids: NS
- Minimize fluids to <500 mL: inc risk of pulmonary edema
- Monitors: std; A-line for open midgestation fetal surgery, Foley
- Fetal hypothermia: room temp 80°

ANESTHETIC PLAN
- Regional: epidural placed as sole anesthetic for fetoscopic cases, and postop analgesia if open hysterotomy
- Induction: RSI: thiopental & sux

- Maintenance: volatile agent >2 MAC for open hysterotomy cases until uterine closure
- Follow with epidural for midgestation surgery or PCA for EXIT procedure
- Epidural only for fetoscopic cases, convert to GETA as needed for additional uterine relaxation
- Emergence: full-dose reversal
- Adjuvant tx: ephedrine to maintain mean BP within 10% of normal; magnesium load at time of uterine closure followed by continuous infusion

PAIN MANAGEMENT
- Systemic: EXIT procedure: PCA
- Regional: open midgestation fetal surgery & fetoscopic cases: PCEA or continuous epidural infusion
- Fentanyl in epidural infusion may provide fetal analgesia

PACU/POSTOPERATIVE CONSIDERATIONS
- Inc risk of preterm labor
- Inc weakness, nausea, lethargy from magnesium

FONTAN PROCEDURE

STEPHEN A. STAYER, MD

CO-EXISTING DISEASES
- Blood diverted from IVC & SVC to PA, bypassing RV
- Blood flow through lung is passive: systemic venous pressure > pulm venous pressure.

PREOPERATIVE ASSESSMENT
- Studies: ECG, CXR, echo, cardiac cath, CBC, lytes, BUN, creat, coags
- Premed: if >1 yr, PO midazolam 0.5 mg/kg; max 15 mg
- NPO: std

PROCEDURAL CONSIDERATIONS

- Supine
- IV fluids: LR, Plasmalyte or Normosol
- Minimize fluids before CPB
- 5% albumin or 6% hetastarch (max 15 mL/kg/24 h) will limit fluids & maintain COP.
- Monitors: std + A-line, CVP
- LA pressure monitored after CBP
- Transesophageal echo std in many centers
- BIS, cerebral oximeter, transcranial Doppler in some centers
- Risks:
- Air embolism: minimize w/ TEE
- Low CO:
  - ➤ Decreased preload: low LA & RA press
  - ➤ Elevated PVR: low LA, high RA press
  - ➤ Obstruction of systemic venous to pulmonary pathway: low LA, high RA press
  - ➤ Myocardial depression: high LA, high RA press
  - ➤ Arrhythmias: loss of AV synchrony decreases CO
- Cyanosis: surgeon commonly places fenestration between systemic venous pathway & LA: allows desaturated blood to fill heart, maintains CO when PVR elevated

ANESTHETIC PLAN

- Inhalation or IV induction
- No myocardial depressants (halothane/thiopental)
- Pts sensitive to higher doses of inhalation agents
- Maintenance: opioids w/ low isoflurane or midazolam
- Avoid N_2O: increases micro-bubbles
- Emergence: pts with good ventricular fn extubated in OR or immed postop
- Pts with limited myocardial reserves stay intubated & ventilated
- Adjuvant tx: Amicar or aprotinin if repeat sternotomy

- Inotropic agents (epinephrine and/or milrinone) & nitroprusside available for pts with low CO
- Occasionally need epicardial pacing
- Rarely NO used to tx pulmonary htn

PAIN MANAGEMENT
- Systemic: see intraop
- Regional: caudal epidural, spinal or thoracic epidural opioids & LAs used; however, controversial since heparinized

PACU/POSTOPERATIVE CONSIDERATIONS
- Mechanical vent with increased intrathoracic press may impair pulmonary blood flow.
- Ventilation w/ low PEEP & adequate exhalation time optimal
- Spontaneous ventilation will improve V/Q match.
- Morphine: intermittent doses, continuous infusion or PCA

FOREIGN BODY IN THE TRACHEA OR BRONCHUS

DAVID A. YOUNG, MD

CO-EXISTING DISEASES
- Respiratory distress, stridor, wheezing
- Location & type of FB determines symptoms
- Atelectasis, pneumonia, hypoxemia
- Contralateral lung contamination
- Peanut: inflammatory response, chemical pneumonitis

PREOPERATIVE ASSESSMENT
- Studies: none required
- Neck X-ray: location, size & shape of FB
- CXR: infiltrate, pneumothorax, atelectasis, mediastinal shift, lung hyperinflation
- Premed: consider IV midazolam 0.05 mg/kg

- Constant monitoring required
- IV glycopyrrolate 0.01 mg/kg or atropine 0.02 mg/kg
- NPO: if stable, delay for 6 h

PROCEDURAL CONSIDERATIONS
- Indeterminate length
- Supine
- IV preferred preop
- IV fluids: any
- Monitors: std
- Risks: laryngospasm, bronchospasm, airway obstruction, airway trauma & edema, barotrauma, hypotension, bleeding, secretions

ANESTHETIC PLAN
- Full stomach premeds:
  - IV ranitidine 1 mg/kg and/or
  - IV metoclopramide 0.1 mg/kg
  - RSI with cricoid pressure
  - Surgeon in OR; all equipment ready
  - Induction option #1: no IV or in resp distress: inhalation (halothane or sevo); 100% O_2; topical lidocaine to larynx (<5 mg/kg)
  - Induction option #2: IV present: TIVA with propofol/remifentanil
  - Spontaneous vs. controlled ventilation: most prefer spont
  - Neither proven superior
  - Spontaneous: may avoid migration of FB; need higher MAC, laryngo/bronchospasm, ventilation self-regulating; ENT sprays topical lidocaine
  - Controlled: prevents bucking & airway trauma, shorter emergence time, easier intubation, potential to push FB farther into bronchus
  - Maintenance: volatile agent in 100% O_2 or propofol/remi infusion with 100% O_2

➤ If complete airway obstruction: mainstem intubation to bypass FB
➤ Once FB removed, check for residual material, edema & secretions
➤ When surgeon finished, intubate with regular ETT & extubate awake
➤ Adjuvant tx: IV dexamethasone 0.5 mg/kg; max 20 mg

PAIN MANAGEMENT
■ Systemic: small-dose IV opioid

PACU/POSTOPERATIVE CONSIDERATIONS
■ Humidified O_2
■ Inspiratory stridor: racemic epi if hypoxemia
■ Expiratory wheeze: nebulized albuterol
■ Analgesia: acetaminophen usually sufficient

FRENULECTOMY

FRANCINE S. YUDKOWITZ, MD, FAAP

CO-EXISTING DISEASES
■ Usually none

PREOPERATIVE ASSESSMENT
■ Studies: none
■ Premed: if >1 yr, PO midazolam 0.5 mg/kg; max 15 mg
■ NPO: std

PROCEDURAL CONSIDERATIONS
■ IV fluids: isotonic crystalloid to replace deficit & maintenance
■ Monitors: std
■ Risks: sharing airway with surgeon
■ May have bleeding into oral cavity

ANESTHETIC PLAN
- Inhalation or IV induction
- Intubation usually not necessary
- Airway management with mask or LMA
- Maintenance: inhalation or TIVA
- Emergence: make sure no bleeding

PAIN MANAGEMENT
- PR acetaminophen 40 mg/kg
- Local anesthetic infiltration

PACU/POSTOPERATIVE CONSIDERATIONS
- None

GASTROSCHISIS REPAIR

RONALD S. LITMAN, DO

CO-EXISTING DISEASES
- More likely than omphalocele to have dehydration, sepsis, & acidosis

PREOPERATIVE ASSESSMENT
- Management of dehydration, sepsis, electrolytes, acidosis
- Studies: hct, lytes, coags, T&C
- Premed: usually none, IV atropine 0.02 mg/kg optional
- NPO since birth
- NG or OG tube in situ

PROCEDURAL CONSIDERATIONS
- Surgeon's main priority is primary repair; limited by high intra-abdominal pressure that causes dec FRC & hypoxemia, IVC compression & hypotension, aorta or renal artery compression & oliguria
- If lesion large, surgeon should place indwelling central venous catheter before repair

- Supine
- IV fluids: glucose maintenance infusion + LR or NS for volume
- Bleeding may be significant & require transfusion
- 3rd space loss at least 20 mL/kg
- Risks: hypoxemia, hypotension, hypoglycemia
- Monitors: std + A-line if lesion large
- 2 good upper extremity IVs or central venous line

ANESTHETIC PLAN

- IV modified RSI; often need ventilation through cricoid pressure
- Unless lesion very small, plan for postop ventilation.
- Maintenance: balanced technique: O_2, air, volatile agent, paralytic, liberal titration of opioid
- Awaken & extubate in OR if lesion very small
- Often need manual bag ventilation during case as surgeon is attempting primary repair
- Constant communication with surgeon is essential; needs to know effects of intra-abdominal contents on SpO_2 & blood pressure
- May need to defer primary repair & place silo for staged repair

PAIN MANAGEMENT

- Systemic: liberal titration of intraop fentanyl
- Regional: caudal epidural catheter can be used intraop and leave in place for postop analgesia

PACU/POSTOPERATIVE CONSIDERATIONS

- Abdominal compartment syndrome: hypoxemia, hypotension, oliguria
- Liberal paralysis if symptomatic
- Analgesia: continue epidural analgesia or opioid infusion

GASTROSTOMY TUBE PLACEMENT

SURESH THOMAS, MD

CO-EXISTING DISEASES
- Neurologic impairment, with compromised ability to swallow & increase risk of aspiration
- Congenital/acquired upper GI tract abnormalities
- Malignancies of head, neck, oral cavity or mediastinum
- Failure to thrive

PREOPERATIVE ASSESSMENT
- Studies: none unless indicated by hx
- Premed: midazolam PO/SC or IV
- Consider H_2 antagonists & metoclopramide
- SBE prophylaxis in at-risk pts
- EMLA cream
- NPO: std

PROCEDURAL CONSIDERATIONS
- Position: Supine
- IV fluids: LR at maintenance after correction of deficits
- Monitors: std
- Risks: aspiration, hypotension (from hypovolemia related to poor intake), bleeding

ANESTHETIC PLAN
- RSI if at risk for aspiration
- Mask or IV induction OK if no aspiration risk
- Maintenance: O_2, air & volatile agent $\pm$ opioids
- In older children: propofol 75–200 mcg/kg/min & fentanyl 1–2 mcg/kg $\pm$ local infiltration
- Awaken & extubate in OR.

PAIN MANAGEMENT

- Systemic: titrate opioid to effect
- Regional: local infiltration by surgeon

PACU/POSTOPERATIVE CONSIDERATIONS

- Analgesia: IV morphine 0.05 mg/kg q5–10 min prn pain
- N/V: consider IV ondansetron 0.1 mg/kg (max 4 mg)

HEART TRANSPLANT

DEAN B. ANDROPOULOS, MD

CO-EXISTING DISEASES

- Dilated cardiomyopathy: viral, idiopathic, chemotherapy, myopathy
- Hypertrophic cardiomyopathy: familial, Noonan syndrome, storage disease
- Congenital heart disease: HLHS, heterotaxy, severe Ebstein's, anomalous L coronary, unbalanced AV canal
- Poor vent function
- AV valve regurgitation
- Shone complex: MS, small LV, LV outflow obstruction, AS, small aortic arch, coarc of aorta
- Failed Fontan

PREOPERATIVE ASSESSMENT

- Studies: CBC, coags, lytes, BUN, creat, LFTs
- CXR, ECG, echo, cath for PVR
- Premed: IV/PO midazolam, IV/PO azathioprine, IV methyl-prednisolone in OR
- NPO: std

PROCEDURAL CONSIDERATIONS

- Supine, roll under shoulders

- IV fluids: LR, 5% albumin for large-volume infusions
- 6% hetastarch in pts >10 yr; max 15 mL/kg/24 h
- Blood products CMV neg, irradiated, leukoreduced
- Std monitors + Foley, A-line, CVP, TEE; maybe PA cath
- Some centers use neuro monitors: BIS, NIRS, transcranial Doppler
- Risks: arrhythmias, hypotension on induction or with positive-press vent; bleeding with repeat sternotomy; pulmonary htn post-CPB; low CO post-CPB; prolonged donor ischemic time > 5 hr; undersized donor; poor donor heart condition; bradycardia post-CPB from denervated heart
- Donor considerations: ABO compatible; body wt 80–160% of recipient; normal cardiac fn by echo; minimal inotropic support

ANESTHETIC PLAN
- IV induction: etomidate, fentanyl, midazolam, vec, roc or pav
- Beware ketamine: myocardial depressant
- Avoid propofol, thiopental, halothane
- Maintenance: fentanyl/midazolam, isoflurane, vec/pav
- Ventilate postop
- Adjuvant tx: Repeat sternotomy: Amicar or aprotinin; NO for pulmonary htn; dopamine for cardiac/renal dysfn; dobutamine/milrinone for inc inotropy or pulmonary htn; isoproterenol for bradycardia in denervated heart; atrial pacing, epi or ECMO/VAD for low CO; external pacing pads for redo sternotomy & high-risk arrhythmia pts

PAIN MANAGEMENT
- Systemic: high-dose opioid

PACU/POSTOPERATIVE CONSIDERATIONS
- Htn if oversized donor: treat with nitroprusside, milrinone
- Early extubation if min bleeding & good myocardial fn

- Analgesia: intermittent opioid, PCA
- Avoid NSAIDs: bleeding risk

HEEL CORD LENGTHENING

JOSEPH D. TOBIAS, MD

CO-EXISTING DISEASES

- Neuromuscular disorders: cerebral palsy (CP), meningomyelocele, muscular dystrophy (MD)
- Global development delay
- Seizure disorder, poor airway control, respiratory muscle weakness
- IF DMD: cardiac involvement, difficulty clearing secretions, GE reflux & risk of aspiration
- Anticonvulsants cause resistance to nondepolarizing NMBAs.
- Hyperkalemia & rhabdomyolysis with succinylcholine & DMD
- Prolonged duration of nondepolarizing NMBAs in DMD
- Possible MH susceptibility

PREOPERATIVE ASSESSMENT

- Studies: if osteotomy: hematocrit, T&S
- Cardiac evaluation (echocardiogram, ECG) if DMD
- Premeds: usual anticonvulsants
- Optional: IV ranitidine 1 mg/kg, max 50 mg; IV metoclopramide 0.15 mg/kg, max 10 mg; PO/GT Bicitra 1 mL/kg, max 30 mL; IV glycopyrrolate 20 µg/kg, max 0.2 mg
- PO/GT midazolam 0.5 mg/kg, max 15 mg in acetaminophen 10–15 mg/kg
- NPO: standard

PROCEDURAL CONSIDERATIONS

- Start prone, sometimes turn supine

- Soft tissue incisions in either Achilles tendon or gastrocnemius
- Often combined with SPLATT (split anterior tibialis tendon transfer)
- Tourniquet may be used.
- IV fluids: warmed LR in upper extremity
- Blood loss if osteotomy
- 3rd space losses: 2–3 mL/kg/h
- BP cuff on upper extremity
- Foley catheter for long procedures
- A-line for bilateral osteotomies, especially if controlled hypotension
- Hypothermia: OR warm until induction complete & pt covered
- Forced warm air during procedure

ANESTHETIC PLAN
- Inhalation induction with sevoflurane or IV with agent of choice
- RSI for severe reflux or inhalation induction with cricoid pressure
- Extubate in OR.

PAIN MANAGEMENT
- IV ketorolac 0.5 mg/kg, max 10 mg
- PO acetaminophen 10–15 mg/kg, PR 40 mg/kg
- Fentanyl 0.5 mcg/kg or morphine 0.02 mg/kg titrated to effect and/or respiratory rate with spontaneous ventilation
- Caudal/lumbar epidural (single-shot or catheter) for bilateral procedures or popliteal fossa block for unilateral procedures.
- Single shot 1 mL/kg of 0.2% ropivacaine, bupivacaine or levobupivacaine; continuous infusion: 0.1% ropivacaine, bupivacaine, levobupivacaine + fentanyl 2.5 mcg/mL at 0.2–0.3 mL/kg/h

PACU/POSTOPERATIVE CONSIDERATIONS

■ Systemic analgesics or regional anesthesia as above

■ Muscle spasms: benzodiazepines & NSAIDs

HYPOSPADIAS REPAIR

PASQUALE DE NEGRI, MD

CO-EXISTING DISEASES

■ None

PREOPERATIVE ASSESSMENT

■ Studies: none

■ Premed: if >1 yr, PO midazolam 0.5 mg/kg; max 15 mg

■ NPO: std

PROCEDURAL CONSIDERATIONS

■ Supine

■ IV fluids: LR at maintenance

■ Very minimal 3rd space loss or bleeding

■ Monitors: std

ANESTHETIC PLAN

■ Inhalation induction with sevoflurane or IV induction with propofol or thiopental

■ NMB of choice to facilitate intubation or if using controlled ventilation

■ ETT or LMA

■ Maintenance: balanced technique: O_2, N_2O, volatile agent

■ Awaken & extubate in OR

PAIN MANAGEMENT

■ Systemic: titrate intraop fentanyl or alfentanil

■ Regional: caudal or penile block (see Circumcision chapter)

PACU/POSTOPERATIVE CONSIDERATIONS
- Analgesia: PR acetaminophen 40 mg/kg, then 20 mg/kg q6h
- PO codeine 0.5–1.0 mg/kg, max 30 mg alone or with acetaminophen

---

IMPERFORATE ANUS REPAIR (PENA PROCEDURE OR POSTERIOR SAGITTAL ANORECTOPLASTY)

RONALD S. LITMAN, DO

CO-EXISTING DISEASES
- Assoc congenital malformations: VACTERL (VATER) syndrome
- Vertebral anomalies involve sacrum: can alter landmarks for placing caudal epidural
- Cardiac lesions: most common VSD
- Tracheoesophageal fistula & esophageal atresia
- Renal/GU malformations
- Limb anomalies
- Procedure usually performed in 1st year of life, as elective procedure when pt healthy

PREOPERATIVE ASSESSMENT
- Studies: none
- Premed: if >1 yr, PO midazolam 0.5 mg/kg; max 10 mg
- NPO: std

PROCEDURAL CONSIDERATIONS
- Usually begins in prone position
- Some surgeons will turn pt & finish supine or lithotomy
- Pt situated at far end of OR table; plan to move after intubation
- IV fluids: warmed LR; 3rd space loss usually 7–10 mL/kg/h
- IV in upper extremity
- Usually little blood loss

- Monitors: std
- Pulse-ox & BP on upper extremities
- Hypothermia: increase temp in OR, forced warm air blanket underneath & around child & HME in breathing circuit

ANESTHETIC PLAN
- Inhalation induction with sevoflurane or IV induction with agent of choice
- NMB may be used to facilitate intubation; no preferred agent.
- ETT required
- Maintenance: balanced technique with O_2, air & volatile agent
- Titrate opioids if no regional.
- Avoid N_2O to prevent bowel distention.
- Awaken pt & extubate trachea at completion of procedure.

PAIN MANAGEMENT
- Systemic: fentanyl preferred
- Morphine, alfentanil, sufentanil & remi acceptable alternatives
- Regional: intraop epidural anesthesia by insertion of catheter via caudal canal after induction of anesthesia & placement of ETT
- Local anesthetic choices: 3% 2-chloroprocaine, 0.15% ropivacaine, or 0.25% bupivacaine

PACU/POSTOPERATIVE CONSIDERATIONS
- Analgesia best accomplished by continuation of epidural meds
- Choices: 2% 2-chloroprocaine, 1.5% lidocaine, or 0.0625-0.125% bupivacaine
- Avoid epidural opioids if <1 yr.
- Systemic: IV morphine 0.05 mg/kg prn

INGUINAL HERNIA REPAIR

ORIGINALLY WRITTEN BY FANNIE SCHAPIRO, MD
REVISED BY RONALD S. LITMAN, DO

CO-EXISTING DISEASES
- More likely to incarcerate in premature infants
- Prematurity & sequelae: RDS, BPD, central apnea, anemia, temp instability, retinopathy
- Incarceration is a surgical emergency: treat as bowel obstruction.

PREOPERATIVE ASSESSMENT
- Studies: hct <6 mo
- Premed: consider midazolam if >8 mo
- NPO: std

PROCEDURAL CONSIDERATIONS
- Supine
- IV fluids: LR; if <1 mo use dextrose-containing solutions
- Monitors: std
- Risks: hypoxia if infant small; vomiting & aspiration if incarcerated

ANESTHETIC PLAN
- Induction: if elective without full stomach, mask induction with sevo + N_2O/O_2 or IV induction with std agents in older child
- If incarcerated, full stomach precautions: RSI & cricoid pressure
- Spinal anesthesia with tetracaine 1 mg/kg with epi wash may be used when appropriate: factors include size of hernia, unilateral vs. bilateral, surgical skill & duration of surgery

- If spinal, try to avoid opioids & sedatives to prevent postop apnea.
- Maintenance: balanced technique: O_2, air & volatile agent
- May use ETT, mask, or LMA
- If spinal: pacifier dipped in glucose useful for comfort
- Local infiltration of hernia sac by surgeon to minimize stimulus during traction
- Awaken & extubate in OR; delayed awakening very common in premature infants; may need to ventilate postop.

PAIN MANAGEMENT
- Titrate opioids if no regional
- Remifentanil ideal
- IV ketorolac 0.5 mg/kg & PR acetaminophen 30 mg/kg
- Regional: as supplement to GA: single-shot caudal with 1 mL/kg 0.125–0.25% bupivacaine after induction
- Field block may be placed at end of surgery.

PACU/POSTOPERATIVE CONSIDERATIONS
- If <55 wk postconceptual age, apnea monitoring for 12–24 h
- Analgesia: acetaminophen/NSAID

INTESTINAL ATRESIA REPAIR

DEBASHISH BHATTACHARYA, MD

CO-EXISTING DISEASES
- Common in duodenum, jejunum & ileum but rare in colon
- Congenital malformations common with duodenal atresia; include Down syndrome, malrotation, esophageal atresia, biliary anomalies, congenital heart disease
- Prematurity (50%)

PREOPERATIVE ASSESSMENT
- Assess for dehydration: weight, pulse, blood pressure, skin turgor, fontanelle, urine output
- Assess respiratory status for aspiration pneumonitis
- Studies: CBC, BUN, bilirubin, glucose, calcium, lytes, T&C, UA with specific gravity
- Not a surgical emergency
- Preoperative hydration & correction of acid-base & electrolyte problems

PROCEDURAL CONSIDERATIONS
- Supine
- IV fluids: D10W or D5/0.2 NaCl for maintenance; LR for replacement
- 2 IVs preferable ± central venous catheter for postop alimentation
- Blood loss usually <10% of blood volume
- 3rd space loss 8–10 mL/kg/h
- Monitors: std + Foley
- A-line if CHD or septicemia
- Warming measures: increase OR temp, radiant & fluid warmers, humidified circuit, warming blanket

ANESTHETIC PLAN
- RSI with sux/atropine or rocuronium
- Maintenance: balanced technique: O_2/air & volatile agent
- Avoid N_2O to prevent bowel distention

PAIN MANAGEMENT
- Titrate opioids: fentanyl 0.5–1 mcg/kg/h

PACU/POSTOPERATIVE CONSIDERATIONS
- Plan to extubate term neonates
- Premies & neonates with assoc anomalies may require postop ventilation.

- Postop analgesia: morphine infusion 10–50 mcg/kg/h
- Regional: caudal epidural catheter may be used if neonate isn't septic

---

INTUSSUSCEPTION REPAIR

CATHY BACHMAN, MD

CO-EXISTING DISEASES
- Bowel obstruction & edema
- Possible ischemia & perforation
- Usually previously healthy
- Abdominal pain, vomiting, blood in stools
- Lethargy, may be obtunded
- Dehydration, sepsis
- Electrolyte disturbances
- Preferred tx: reduction with barium enema under radiology guidance
- Surgery if reduction unsuccessful or if peritoneal signs or free air in abdomen

PREOPERATIVE ASSESSMENT
- Studies: H/H, lytes
- Premed: none; atropine optional
- Sedative usually not needed: pts often lethargic
- NPO: treat as full stomach

PROCEDURAL CONSIDERATIONS
- Supine
- IV fluids: NS or LR resuscitation & maintenance
- 10–15 mL/kg/h for 3rd space
- Std monitors ± Foley
- Risks: aspiration on induction, hypotension, hypovolemia, sepsis & hypothermia

ANESTHETIC PLAN
- Fluid resuscitation before induction
- RSI & endotracheal intubation
- Maintenance: balanced technique: oxygen and air & volatile agent
- Avoid nitrous oxide.
- Titrate opioids if no regional technique used.
- Awake extubation in OR

PAIN MANAGEMENT
- Systemic: titrate opioid
- Regional: single-shot caudal: 0.25% bupivacaine 1 mL/kg +/− additive
- Indwelling epidural catheter: 0.1% bupivacaine + appropriate dose of opioid if >3 months

PACU/POSTOPERATIVE CONSIDERATIONS
- Fluid & electrolyte balance, pain mgmt, possible sepsis
- Titrate IV opioids if no regional.
- Epidural infusion with local anesthetic alone or local anesthetic/opioid combo
- Same infusion doses as for intraop

KASAI PROCEDURE FOR BILIARY ATRESIA

GREGORY S. CAMBIER, MD AND PETER J. DAVIS, MD

CO-EXISTING DISEASES
- Polysplenia syndrome: situs inversus, absent IVC, cardiac defects, anomalous hepatic artery supply; intestinal malrotation
- Direct hyperbilirubinemia during 1–6 wk of life
- Procedure performed by 4 mo

PREOPERATIVE ASSESSMENT
- Studies: H/H, coags, LFTs, T&C
- Premed: vitamin K 1 mg qd × 4d before surgery
- NPO: std

PROCEDURAL CONSIDERATIONS
- Supine
- IV fluids: warmed LR, 3rd space loss 6–10 mL/kg/h
- If venous access a problem, central line may be needed.
- If hypoglycemia occurs, add dextrose to IV fluids.
- Monitors: std + Foley, forced warm air blanket, A-line dependent on coexisting disease
- Risks: delayed metabolism of drugs, hypothermia, bleeding, infection, hypothermia

ANESTHETIC PLAN
- Inhalation induction with sevo or halothane; IV induction with agent of choice
- NMB: facilitates intubation & improves vision of surgical site
- Cisatracurium preferred: lack of hepatic metabolism
- ETT required
- Maintenance: balanced technique: O_2, air & volatile agent
- Titrate opioid of choice.
- Avoid N_2O to prevent bowel distention.
- Awaken & extubate in OR.
- Prevent hypothermia.

PAIN MANAGEMENT
- Opioids if regional unavailable
- Systemic: fentanyl 1–2 mcg/kg/dose
- Morphine 0.05–0.10 mg/kg/dose
- Regional OK but coagulopathy risk factors may be present
- Regional: intraop & postop caudal epidural analgesia, if no underlying coagulopathy

- 0.25% bupivacaine intraop & 0.05–0.1% postop/ropivacaine 0.2% intraop & 0.05–0.2% postop

PACU/POSTOPERATIVE CONSIDERATIONS
- Caudal catheter with local anesthetics for postop pain control
- Systemic opioids: morphine 0.05–0.1 mg/kg prn

KIDNEY TRANSPLANT

SCOTT D. MARKOWITZ, MD

CO-EXISTING DISEASES
- Hypertension, CHF, uremia (pericarditis, platelet dysfn), cardiomyopathy, increased intravascular volume & CO, hyperkalemia, hyperphosphatemia, hypocalcemia, hypermagnesemia, metabolic acidosis
- Alagille's syndrome: liver & cardiac anomalies
- Dec protein & inc volume of distribution alter drug action

PREOPERATIVE ASSESSMENT
- Studies: H&H, lytes
- Premed: if >1 yr, PO midazolam 0.3 mg/kg; max 10 mg
- Hemodialysis corrects electrolyte abnormalities, reduces intravascular volume & may improve platelet fn
- NPO: std; uremia: delayed gastric emptying

PROCEDURAL CONSIDERATIONS
- Supine
- Abdominal organ placement for infants, pelvic for older children
- IV fluids: warmed NS/albumin as required for CVP 12–18
- Keep hgb ≥9 g/dL
- Volume load before unclamping
- Monitors: std + CVP

- A-line if aortic cross-clamp
- Risks: hyperkalemia, hypothermia with reperfusion, hemorrhage, oliguria

ANESTHETIC PLAN
- Induction: thiopental, cisatracurium or sux for RSI (if K < 5.5), fentanyl
- Maintenance: isoflurane, monitor NMB with nerve stimulator
- Awaken & extubate in OR
- Replace urine output (may be large volume if adult-sized donor kidney)
- Adjuvant tx: heparin before cross-clamping
- Cefazolin/gentamicin preop
- Immunosuppression with thymoglobulin (premed with acetaminophen and diphenhydramine and Solu-Medrol) or basiliximab (2 hours prior to transplant) or daclizumab
- Mannitol 0.25–0.5 g/kg & furosemide 1 mg/kg before unclamping
- Fresh or washed RBCs
- May need albumin, calcium or dopamine for reperfusion hypotension

PAIN MANAGEMENT
- Systemic: morphine is preferred, hydromorphone or fentanyl for postop renal dysfunction or intolerance to morphine
- Morphine can lead to respiratory depression.
- Normeperidine may accumulate in renal failure. Avoid NSAIDs.

PACU/POSTOPERATIVE CONSIDERATIONS
- Analgesia: IV opioid/PCA
- Pt may continue to need dialysis postop for short time.
- Urine output volume should be replaced to avoid hypovolemia (keep CVP 12–15).

LACRIMAL DUCT PROBING & IRRIGATION

PETE G. KOVATSIS, MD

CO-EXISTING DISEASES
- Usually none

PREOPERATIVE ASSESSMENT
- Studies: none
- Premed: weigh against brevity of procedure
- PO/PR midazolam 0.5 mg/kg
- Acetaminophen 10–20 mg/kg PO
- NPO: std

PROCEDURAL CONSIDERATIONS
- Supine
- Ophthalmologist probes & irrigates lacrimal duct to verify patency.
- Surgical stimulation mild
- IV recommended: see risks
- Monitors: std
- Risks: Oculocardiac reflex due to pressure on globe; results in bradycardia; laryngospasm
- Irrigation fluid may pass into pharynx via the nasal passages & cause laryngospasm if pt in light plane of anesthesia.
- May use nasal suction during irrigation to decrease fluid into larynx

ANESTHETIC PLAN
- Std inhalation or IV induction
- Use face mask or LMA.
- ETT only if dictated by clinical scenario
- Maintenance: inhalation agent in O_2/N_2O with spontaneous vent

- Maintain adequate depth of anesthesia until irrigation completed.
- Suction pharynx if large amount of irrigation required.
- Awaken in OR.

PAIN MANAGEMENT
- Acetaminophen

PACU/POSTOPERATIVE CONSIDERATIONS
- Analgesia: continue acetaminophen and/or nonsteroidal

LAPAROSCOPY

DARRYL BERKOWITZ, MD

CO-EXISTING DISEASES
- Any intra-abdominal process

PREOPERATIVE ASSESSMENT
- Std fasting & premed
- Labs: T&C for neonates/infants

PROCEDURAL CONSIDERATIONS
- Neonatal/infant viscera & blood vessels may be punctured with blind insufflation.
- CO_2 absorption across peritoneal cavity with increased CO_2 elimination
- Hypercarbia will stimulate SNS with tachycardia, hypertension & arrhythmias.
- Increased intra-abdominal pressure (IAP) leads to reduced FRC, increased airway pressure, decreased compliance.
- Trendelenburg position & GA will cause VQ mismatch; not well tolerated because FRC low & baseline O_2 consumption high, leading to hypoxia
- <4 months of age: IAP <6 mmHg because of effects on PVR & potential for reversal of intracardiac shunt

- Infants: keep IAP <10; if higher, increased SVR, decreased CO + SV with MAP remaining unchanged, BUT if keep < 6, then all parameters near normal (this is also found in young children <6 years of age)
- Increased ICP from CO_2 absorption, Trendelenburg, increased intrathoracic pressure & increased IVC pressure (increased intrathecal pressure and decreased CSF absorption)
- Decreased GFR/decreased UO, even if prehydrated; will resolve when pneumoperitoneum gone
- Temperature: hypothermia from CO_2 insufflation

ANESTHETIC PLAN
- Std monitors unless comorbidities
- Std inhalation or IV induction agents; RSI if full stomach
- ETT required
- Maintenance: O_2/Air/Volatile or TIVA
- Warm humidified gases, warm fluid, warm OR
- Need adequate ventilation to overcome hypercarbia from intraperitoneal CO_2 absorption
- Positioning changes frequent to facilitate surgical visibility
- IV catheters above diaphragm in case of IVC compression
- Orogastric tube to drain stomach
- Antiemetic: ondansetron/dexamethasone
- PEEP: to counteract effect of increased IAP on lung bases, causing atelectasis
- Vigilance keeping IAP low
- Emergence: abdominal cavity evacuated, awake extubation
- Complications: unintentional visceral penetration
- CO_2 effects: subcutaneous emphysema, pneumothorax, pneumomediastinum, hypercapnia, gas embolism

PAIN MANAGEMENT
- Intraop: IV opioid, rectal acetaminophen, local anesthetic, IV NSAID
- Postop: any narcotic

PACU/POSTOPERATIVE CONSIDERATIONS

- Residual intraperitoneal CO_2 may cause impairment of ventilation, nausea, shoulder pain.
- PONV common; difficult to treat without prophylaxis

LASER REMOVAL OF PORT WINE STAIN

RONALD S. LITMAN, DO

CO-EXISTING DISEASES

- Sturge-Weber syndrome: angiomatosis involving brain & other organ systems causing seizures, hemiparesis, cognitive & developmental dysfunction, glaucoma
- Klippel-Trenaunay syndrome: vascular malformations of lower limbs causing hypertrophy or atrophy; rare hematuria, anemia, thrombocytopenia, high-output CHF

PREOPERATIVE ASSESSMENT

- Studies: none except if pt has known coexisting disease
- Premed: if >1 yr, midazolam 0.5 mg/kg PO; max 10 mg
- NPO: std

PROCEDURAL CONSIDERATIONS

- Supine; OR table may be turned 90° or away from side of face involved
- Procedure involves laser to face to lighten color of lesion
- All usual laser precautions (eg, wet gauze over pt's eyes)
- IV fluids: LR; 3rd space loss minimal
- Monitors: std
- Risks: hyperthermia from overuse of warming devices

ANESTHETIC PLAN

- Inhalation induction with sevoflurane or IV agent of choice
- NMB of choice may be used to facilitate intubation.

- Keep flammability minimal by avoiding N_2O & maintain low FIO_2.
- ETT or LMA usually required
- Maintenance: balanced technique with air, O_2 & volatile agent
- Awaken & extubate in OR

PAIN MANAGEMENT
- Systemic: titrate intraop fentanyl or morphine
- IV ketorolac 0.5 mg/kg
- Regional: none

PACU/POSTOPERATIVE CONSIDERATIONS
- Pain can be severe: opioids titrated to comfort, PR acetaminophen 40 mg/kg in OR then 20 mg/kg q6h or PO ibuprofen 10 mg/kg q6h
- PO oxycodone 0.1 mg/kg

LIVER TRANSPLANT

J. LANCE LICHTOR, MD

CO-EXISTING DISEASES
- Portal htn, variceal hemorrhage, hypersplenism, thrombocytopenia, ascites
- Pulmonary dysfn: dec lung volumes, pleural effusions, hepatosplenomegaly
- Intrapulmonary R-to-L shunt through dilated pulmonary arterioles
- Impaired hypoxic pulmonary vasoconstriction & pulmonary diffusion
- Cardiac dysfn: hyperdynamic circ & low SVR, renal vasoconstriction, poor clearance of vasoactive substances, A–V shunting, tissue hypoxia

PREOPERATIVE ASSESSMENT
- Studies: T&C, CBC, lytes, coags
- NPO: std if not urgent

PROCEDURAL CONSIDERATIONS
- Phase 1: skin incision, liver dissection, vessel clamping
- Phase 2: removal of liver, insert new liver
- Phase 3: reperfusion of new liver
- IV fluids: LR; 3rd space loss 12–15 mL/kg/h
- Blood loss usually <1 BV but may be up to 10 BVs
- Monitors: std; pulse ox & BP on UEs; Foley, A-line, CVP and in some institutions SG catheter
- Risks: hypothermia; forced warm air blanket, warm peritoneal lavage
- Blood & fluid loss in phase 1
- Avoid excess fluid in phase 2: CV failure with liver reperfusion
- Circ disturbances in phase 3 from effluent from new liver (high K, low pH & temp); possible infusion of air or microthrombi into heart: pulmonary htn, bradycardia, ventricular dysrhythmias, arrest
- Flushing of new liver with colloid then retrograde flushing with recipient blood decreases K & pH problems.
- Split allografts allow 1 donor liver for 2 pts
- Monitor pH & glucose q1h in phases 1 & 3, q30 min in phase 2
- Hypoglycemia in phases 1 & 2
- Venous bypass not used if pt <20 kg; without venous bypass lower body venous engorgement, oliguria & intestinal complications more common
- Oversized allograft may lead to ventilation diff when abdomen closed

ANESTHETIC PLAN
- Induction: no pref; NMB OK (do not over-paralyze since occasionally case cancelled after abdomen opened), RSI if full stomach

■ Maintenance: balanced technique: O_2, air, isoflurane or desflurane

■ Adjuvant tx: dopamine prn; immunosuppression varies by institution

PAIN MANAGEMENT

■ Systemic: any opioid

■ Regional: consider thoracic epidural if no coagulopathy

PACU/POSTOPERATIVE CONSIDERATIONS

■ <24 h: clot evacuation

■ >24 h: biliary leak, abscess drainage, liver bx, graft vessel occlusion

■ Large 3rd space fluid loss

■ Met alkalosis from bicarb, citrate in blood, diuretics & NG drainage

---

LOWER EXTREMITY FRACTURE

SAM SHARAR, MD

CO-EXISTING DISEASES

■ Other injuries: head, abdomen, thorax

■ Hypovolemia from blood loss

PREOPERATIVE ASSESSMENT

■ Studies: hct

■ Premed: IV midazolam $\pm$ opioids

■ NPO: std; usually considered full stomach

PROCEDURAL CONSIDERATIONS

■ Usually supine; prone or lateral for some pelvis, hip, femur fractures

■ IV fluids: replace with warmed LR & RBC; blood products guided by BP, HR, urine output, serial hcts

- Fluid requirements higher with pelvis & femur fractures due to occult blood loss & possible assoc injuries (eg, liver, spleen)
- IV access in upper extremities to avoid op sites & tourniquets
- Monitors: std + Foley
- Risks: hypothermia (exposure, fluid replacement): inc room temp, use fluid warmers & upper body forced air blanket

ANESTHETIC PLAN

- RSI with etomidate (if hypovolemia) or thiopental/propofol (if normovolemia) & sux or roc
- If elective: mask sevo or IV induction
- Often need NMB to facilitate fx reduction or positioning
- ETT required if emergent surgery (aspiration risk); ETT/LMA for elective surgery
- Maintenance: balanced technique: O_2, N_2O, volatile agent
- Avoid N_2O if risk/presence of assoc thoracic injury or pneumothorax.
- Awaken & extubate in OR.

PAIN MANAGEMENT

- Systemic: titrate fentanyl or hydromorphone or morphine
- Regional block: caudal, epidural, sciatic/femoral for postop pain, only in normovolemic pts with isolated extremity fractures: risk of hypotension with sympathectomy + hypovolemia
- Discuss with surgeon risks of compartment syndrome prior to regional.

PACU/POSTOPERATIVE CONSIDERATIONS

- Analgesia: systemic opioids, regional
- PCA in appropriate pts
- Continuous neurovascular assessment to identify compartment syndrome

LUNG TRANSPLANT

DEAN B. ANDROPOULOS, MD

CO-EXISTING DISEASES

- Cystic fibrosis: hyperinflation, obstruction, secretions, infection
- Primary pulmonary hypertension: prostacyclin infusion
- Bronchopulmonary dysplasia
- Irreparable cardiac: VSD & Eisenmenger's physiology

PREOPERATIVE ASSESSMENT

- Studies: CBC, coags, lytes, BUN, creat, LFTs
- ECG, echo, cath for PVR
- Premed: IV/PO midazolam, IV/PO azathioprine, IV methylprednisolone in OR
- NPO: std

PROCEDURAL CONSIDERATIONS

- Single lung transplant (SLT) or bilateral sequential SLT (most children), or
- Double lung, living related donor lobar transplant (2 donors, 1 lobe each), or
- Heart-lung transplant: en bloc technique
- Supine: arms at side for median sternotomy
- Arms suspended on ether screen for clamshell thoracosternotomy incision
- Lat decub for thoracotomy for SLT
- IV fluids: LR, 5% albumin for large-volume infusions
- 6% hetastarch in pts > 10 yr; max 15 mL/kg/24 h
- Blood products CMV neg, leukoreduced, irradiated
- Monitors: std + Foley, A-line, CVP
- PA line if pulmonary htn
- Maybe SvO_2, RVEF, TEE

- Some centers use neuro monitors: BIS, NIRS, transcranial Doppler
- Donor: ABO compatible, close size match with recipient, minimal lung disease
- Risks: pulmonary htn, RV failure, post-reperfusion pulmonary edema, obstructed pulmonary veins, pneumothorax, hypoxemia, disparate lung compliance, coagulopathy
- Limit donor ischemic time < 6–8 h

ANESTHETIC PLAN

- IV induction: etomidate, fentanyl, midazolam, vec, roc or panc
- Beware ketamine: myocardial depressant
- Avoid propofol, thiopental, halothane
- OLV used in larger pts or for SLT
- DLT if >25–30 kg
- Smaller pts: mainstem intubation with regular small cuffed ETT, or Univent ETT, or bronchial blocker: Fogarty or Arndt
- If CPB, conventional ETT
- Maintenance: high-dose fentanyl/midazolam, low-dose isoflurane, vec or panc
- Ventilate postop
- Adjuvant tx: NO if pulmonary htn, aprotinin if coagulopathy

PAIN MANAGEMENT

- Systemic: opioids
- No regional if heparinized; consider immed postop if not bleeding

PACU/POSTOPERATIVE CONSIDERATIONS

- Minimize crystalloid.
- Give diuretics to reduce lung water.
- Analgesia: opioids; PCA in appropriate pts
- Avoid NSAIDs: bleeding

MEDIASTINOSCOPY

RONALD S. LITMAN, DO

CO-EXISTING DISEASES

- Mediastinal mass: usually lymphoma
- Procedure performed for biopsy or excision of mass

PREOPERATIVE ASSESSMENT

- Studies: hct, T&S, WBC & plts if leukemia
- Premed: if 1 yr, midazolam 0.5 mg/kg PO; max 10 mg; avoid if pre-op respiratory symptoms present
- NPO: std
- Must determine extent of tracheal compression by mass: symptoms of tracheal compression include coughing or dyspnea when supine.
- Review CXR & chest CT to look for tracheal and/or great vessel compression.
- If tracheal and/or great vessel compression, risk of complete obstruction and death on induction of GA: therefore, do case only if necessary

PROCEDURAL CONSIDERATIONS

- Supine
- IV fluids: LR; 3rd space loss 3–6 mL/kg/h
- Monitors: std
- Pulse ox on R hand to detect brachiocephalic artery compression
- Rigid bronch in OR on standby with surgeon present in case life-threatening compression occurs

ANESTHETIC PLAN

- If no tracheal or vessel compression, IV or inhalation induction & NMB of choice
- If tracheal or vessel compression, inhalation induction in semi-sitting position & keep spontaneous ventilation to

maintain negative intrathoracic pressure & avoid further compression

- Intubate during spontaneous ventilation: can push ETT past tracheal compression if necessary
- May require rigid bronchoscopy if obstruction below carina
- If obstruction still not relieved, turn pt lateral or prone to take pressure off trachea or great vessels.
- Last resorts: emergency thoracotomy or initiation of CPB
- Maintenance: balanced technique: O_2, N_2O, isoflurane
- Awaken & extubate in OR

PAIN MANAGEMENT

- Systemic: titrate fentanyl
- Regional: none

PACU/POSTOPERATIVE CONSIDERATIONS

- Analgesia: opioids usually not necessary
- IV ketorolac 0.5 mg/kg/dose q6h
- CXR to R/O pneumothorax

MRI

RONALD S. LITMAN, DO

CO-EXISTING DISEASES

- CNS lesions, peripheral masses

PREOPERATIVE ASSESSMENT

- Studies: none
- Premed: if nec, PO midazolam 0.5 mg/kg, max 10 mg
- Consider parent present during induction
- NPO: std
- Turn off programmable vagal stims
- Possible X-RAY of VP shunt

PROCEDURAL CONSIDERATIONS

- Supine but lateral acceptable for most brain scans

- Pt not within reach during scan
- IV fluids: any
- Monitors: special MRI monitors required
- Pt trauma possible from ferromagnetic objects as projectile missiles
- Hypothermia possible in infants

ANESTHETIC PLAN
- Inhaled or IV induction
- Anesthesiologist can stay inside or outside scanner.
- Airway mgmt depends on clinical situation & anesthesiologist pref: ETT, LMA, oral/nasal airway, or nasal cannula
- Maintenance: TIVA or inhalational
- TIVA (propofol 200 mcg/kg/min) if anesthesia machine unavailable
- Controlled ventilation if MR-safe ventilator present
- Mild upper airway obstruction may result in pt movement & MRI artifact.
- Proactively determine plan for emergence either at scanner or PACU.

PAIN MANAGEMENT
- None

PACU/POSTOPERATIVE CONSIDERATIONS
- None

MRI AND CT SCANS

YVON F. BRYAN, MD

CO-EXISTING DISEASES
- Can have any coexisting disease
- Pts with metallic objects in their body excluded from MRI

PREOPERATIVE ASSESSMENT

■ Studies: none
■ Premed: depends on age & anxiety
■ Consider parent present during induction
■ NPO: std

PROCEDURAL CONSIDERATIONS

■ Supine
■ Pt not within reach
■ May have to interrupt study to assess pt's condition
■ IV fluids: any
■ Monitors: std
■ MRI-safe nonferromagnetic equipment required
■ Risks: tragic accidents due to ferromagnetic objects as projectile missiles & pt injury

ANESTHETIC PLAN

■ Inhaled induction for young children with or without sedation
■ In CT, anesthesiologist can stay either inside or outside scanner.
■ Airway mgmt variable; depends on clinical situation & prefs of anesthesiologist: ETT, LMA, oral/nasal airway, or no airway device all OK
■ Maintenance: choices numerous
■ Find right blend with regard to pt's dx, equipment available & comfort level of personnel
■ TIVA necessary if anesthesia machine unavailable: propofol ideal, 200 mcg/kg/min
■ Rarely need additional meds
■ Another option: spontaneous vent with inhalational agent via LMA/ETT
■ Controlled ventilation if MR-safe ventilator present
■ IV sedation with benzodiazepines or barbiturates possible
■ Inform technicians if need to interrupt study for pt movement, physiologic change, or monitor artifacts

- May allow parent inside scanner
- Emergence: decide whether to extubate awake or deep, inside scanner or in PACU
- If outside scanner, have all monitors & equipment on hand.
- Adjuvant tx: ear plugs or headphones with music to decrease scanner noise

PAIN MANAGEMENT
- None required

PACU/POSTOPERATIVE CONSIDERATIONS
- Proactively determine plan for emergence either at scanner facility or remote PACU

MYELOMENINGOCELE REPAIR

ORIGINALLY WRITTEN BY PEDRO P. VANZILLOTA, MD
REVISED BY RONALD S. LITMAN, DO

CO-EXISTING DISEASES
- Shunt-dependent hydrocephalus: Arnold-Chiari type II malformation; clinically significant in 70–80% after defect closure

PREOPERATIVE ASSESSMENT
- Studies: hct, glucose
- NPO: std

PROCEDURAL CONSIDERATIONS
- Repair usually within 24 h of birth
- Prone, with pads for head & neck to allow chest & abdomen excursion during ventilation & venous return through IVC
- ETT & eyelids securely taped

- Need access to inspect ETT, circuit connections & possible eye compression
- IV fluids: warmed LR at maintenance + 6–8 mL/kg/h; attention to large potential 3rd space loss
- Glucose to correct confirmed hypoglycemia
- Blood loss minimal unless undermining of skin and/or rotation of myocutaneous flaps required
- Blood available from beginning of procedure
- Monitors: std
- Risks: hypothermia; increase temp in OR, forced warm air blanket underneath & around pt
- Latex precautions

ANESTHETIC PLAN
- Induction & intubation in lateral position or supine with cushioned ring around defect
- Inhalation or IV induction
- ETT required
- Maintenance: controlled ventilation mandatory to prevent hypoventilation & hypercarbia
- Fentanyl preferred to ensure wakefulness at completion
- Avoid long-acting NMBs.
- Awaken & extubate in OR or shortly afterward.

PAIN MANAGEMENT
- Systemic: fentanyl
- Regional: usually none; spinal anesthesia possible by surgeon applying tetracaine to CSF over lesion
- Local infiltration with bupivacaine or ropivacaine 2–3 mg/kg at end of surgery

PACU/POSTOPERATIVE CONSIDERATIONS
- Central apnea

MYRINGOTOMY & TUBES INSERTION

JENNIFER MOGAN, MD

CO-EXISTING DISEASES
- Eustachian tube dysfunction due to congenital obstruction or adenotonsillar hypertrophy
- Concurrent URI common

PREOPERATIVE ASSESSMENT
- Studies: none
- Premed: best avoided since procedure short; midazolam for anxious child
- NPO: std

PROCEDURAL CONSIDERATIONS
- Supine: head turned lateral; may cause upper airway obstruction
- IV unnecessary unless indicated
- Monitors: std
- Preop SpO_2 in children with URI
- Risks: laryngospasm possible if adequate depth of anesthesia not achieved before myringotomy

ANESTHETIC PLAN
- Induction: mask induction with O_2, N_2O & sevo
- Maintenance: sevo
- Short procedure, usually ~10 min
- Consider oral airway: nasal passages often obstructed
- Emergence: rapid if procedure short

PAIN MANAGEMENT
- Systemic: intraop nasal fentanyl 1–2 mcg/kg (laryngospasm possible if adequate depth of anesthesia not achieved prior

to administration) provides analgesia & decreases agitation at emergence

- Acetaminophen 10–15 mg/kg PO preop, or acetaminophen 30–40 mg/kg PR post-induction
- Regional: topical anesthesia using EMLA cream can successfully be used in laser-assisted myringotomy in place of general anesthesia in older children

PACU/POSTOPERATIVE CONSIDERATIONS

- Analgesia: pain after procedure is present on awakening & subsides after 45–60 minutes
- Analgesia described above provides adequate pain control on emergence & pt can be sent home with prn ibuprofen or acetaminophen.
- Concurrent URI may increase risk of postoperative airway problems.
- Children with concurrent URI should be given supplemental O_2 to maintain SpO_2 >93%.

NECROTIZING ENTEROCOLITIS (NEC)

RICHARD ROWE, MD, MPH

CO-EXISTING DISEASES

- Sepsis, coagulopathy, respiratory insufficiency, metabolic & respiratory acidosis, shock, hypoglycemia, CHF, PDA, hypothermia

PREOPERATIVE ASSESSMENT

- Studies: CBC, lytes, glucose, coags, recent blood gas helpful
- Premed: usually none
- NPO: full stomach

PROCEDURAL CONSIDERATIONS

- Monitors: std + A-line, CVP helpful but access often difficult

- Foley not routine in neonate
- IV fluids: LR or NS
- 3rd space > 10 mL/kg/h
- If coagulopathy, fresh whole blood, packed RBCs, FFP, plts
- Continue hyperal at maint rate
- Risks: dehydration from underestimating 3rd space loss
- Do not overtransfuse: risk CHF
- Replace RBCs slowly: rapid transfusion will decrease calcium
- Correct coagulopathy with FFP & platelets
- Metabolic acidosis: treat BE < −10 with slow admin of bicarb
- Respiratory acidosis: RR 60–90, VT 10–15 mL/kg, may require HFV
- Maintain PaO_2 60–80
- Hypercarbia: maintain $PaCO_2$ 40–60
- Decrease ETT dead space with side-sampling $ETCO_2$ adapter
- Anemia: keep hct in 30s
- Hypoglycemia: keep glucose 60–100
- Adjust IV fluid to maintain normal lytes: neonate unable to concentrate or dilute urine
- Hypotension: ensure normovolemia
- Stressed neonate may require pressor: dopamine 5–20 mcg/kg/min
- Hypothermia: maintain normal temp with forced air warmer, IV fluid warmer, increase room temp
- Sepsis: antibiotics

ANESTHETIC PLAN

- Induction: if pt stable: RSI with propofol 2–4 mg/kg or pentothal 4–6 mg/kg
- NMB: sux 2 mg/kg or roc 2 mg/kg
- Correct hypotension before RSI or use IV ketamine 1–2 mg/kg
- Awake intubation not preferred in neonate, but depends on skills of practitioner

- Atropine before intubation if using sux
- Maintenance: air, O_2, fentanyl, isoflurane; avoid N_2O
- Place OG or NG tube
- Pt intubated postop

PAIN MANAGEMENT
- Systemic: titrate fentanyl (or analog) to hemodynamics
- Regional not used because concern of sepsis, coagulopathy

PACU/POSTOPERATIVE CONSIDERATIONS
- High risk of significant 3rd space losses, coagulopathy, sepsis, acidosis, hypoglycemia, CHF

NISSEN FUNDOPLICATION

FRANCINE S. YUDKOWITZ, MD, FAAP

CO-EXISTING DISEASES
- GERD
- Pts usually neuro impaired
- Pulmonary disease: recurrent aspiration

PREOPERATIVE ASSESSMENT
- Assess & optimize resp status
- Studies: T&H; hct if suspect anemia
- Other labs based on comorbidity
- Premeds: consider Bicitra 15–30 mL PO, metoclopramide 0.15 mg/kg IV, cimetidine 5–10 mg/kg IV, ranitidine 0.5–1 mg/kg IV, or famotidine 0.3–0.4 mg/kg IV
- NPO: full stomach protocol

PROCEDURAL CONSIDERATIONS
- Open or laparoscopic
- IV fluids: isotonic crystalloid to replace deficit & maintenance

- If open procedure 6–7 mL/kg/h
- If laparoscopy 3–4 mL/kg/h
- Usually minimal blood loss
- Monitors: std
- A-line if pulmonary disease
- Esophageal bougie inserted by anesthesiologist to prevent excessive narrowing of esophagus
- Laparoscopy: intraabdominal pressure < 12 mmHg
- Risks: pneumothorax, visceral trauma, hemorrhage, vena cava compression, laceration
- Air embolus during laparoscopy

ANESTHETIC PLAN
- RSI with cricoid pressure
- Pts with bronchospasm should have adequate depth of anesthesia before intubation.
- Maintenance: no technique preferable
- Avoid N_2O in laparoscopy.
- NMBs should be used.
- Increase minute ventilation: $ETCO_2$ will increase secondary to insufflation of abdomen with CO_2
- Extubate awake unless pulmonary or neuro disease

PAIN MANAGEMENT
- Systemic: intraop opioids
- Morphine avoided in pts with bronchospasm
- Less analgesics with laparoscopy

PACU/POSTOPERATIVE CONSIDERATIONS
- Analgesia: IV fentanyl 1–2 mcg/kg/dose or IV morphine 0.1 mg/kg/dose
- Respiratory compromise in pts with significant pulmonary disease
- Vomiting impaired: intestinal obstruction is emergency

NORWOOD STAGE 1 PROCEDURE

SUANNE DAVES, MD

CO-EXISTING DISEASES

- Initial palliation for infants with hypoplastic L heart syndrome (HLHS) or hypoplastic aortic arch
- Provides relief of systemic outflow obstruction (aortic arch augmentation), adequate mixing (atrial septectomy) & restriction/control of pulmonary blood flow (via BT shunt)

PREOPERATIVE ASSESSMENT

- Preserve ductal patency with PGE1 infusion.
- Maintain balanced pulmonary & systemic blood flow ratio (Qp:Qs). May require controlled ventilation, hypercapnia, inotropes.
- Search for evidence of poor systemic perfusion (Qp > Qs): metabolic acidosis, rising lactate, poor peripheral pulses, mottling, poor urine output.

PROCEDURAL CONSIDERATIONS

- Right upper extremity A-line advantageous if regional low-flow perfusion (RLFP) anticipated for arch reconstruction: umbilical or femoral arterial line vs NIBP on leg allows assessment of residual aortic arch gradient
- Maintain PGE1 infusion until onset of CPB.
- Before CPB, pulmonary overcirculation (Qp > Qs) may be temporarily corrected by surgeon partially occluding branch Pas.
- Deep hypothermic circulatory arrest vs RLFP may be used for arch reconstruction.
- Consider antifibrinolytics.
- Extensive aortic suture lines make restoration of effective hemostasis challenging.

ANESTHETIC PLAN

- Strict attention to PVR/SVR balance (balanced Qp:Qs)
- Vent maneuvers that lower PVR (O_2 therapy and/or hyperventilation) could lead to CV collapse.
- Induction with ketamine/narcotic
- NMB to facilitate intubation
- TEE not generally helpful
- Maintenance: opioid-based
- Myocardial depression with volatile agents possible
- Weaning from CPB: ventilation & oxygenation to maintain Qp:Qs at 0.5 to 1
- If Qp > Qs, vent maneuvers to raise PVR vs afterload reduction
- If Qp: Qs < 0.5, vent measures to lower PVR, seek factors that may elevate PVR (hemo- or pneumothorax, hypercarbia, hypoxemia)
- Afterload reduction, inotropes & bicarb administration may be required to balance PVR/SVR.
- BT shunt may need to be resized if above strategies fail to achieve near-balanced circulation.

PAIN MANAGEMENT

- Continuous opioids

PACU/POSTOPERATIVE CONSIDERATIONS

- Sedation, neuromuscular blockade & mechanical ventilation
- Maintain balanced Qp:Qs.
- Anticipate falling PVR postop.

OMPHALOCELE REPAIR

RONALD S. LITMAN, DO

CO-EXISTING DISEASES

- Hypoglycemia

- Beckwith-Wiedemann syndrome: macroglossia, visceromegaly & renal medulla dysplasia
- Lung disease if premature

PREOPERATIVE ASSESSMENT
- Studies: hct, lytes, coags, T&C
- Premed: none; atropine optional
- NPO: consider full stomach; should have NG or OG tube in situ

PROCEDURAL CONSIDERATIONS
- Surgeon's main priority is primary repair; limited by high intraabdominal pressure that causes dec FRC & hypoxemia, IVC compression & hypotension, aorta or renal artery compression & oliguria
- If lesion large, surgeon should place indwelling central venous catheter before repair.
- Supine
- IV fluids: LR with glucose maintenance infusion (prone to hypoglycemia)
- Bleeding may be significant, requiring transfusion.
- 3rd space loss >20 mL/kg
- Risks: hypoxemia, hypotension, hypoglycemia
- Monitors: std + A-line if lesion large
- 2 good upper extremity IVs or central venous line

ANESTHETIC PLAN
- IV modified RSI; often need ventilation
- Unless lesion very small, plan for postop ventilation.
- Maintenance: balanced technique: O_2, air, inhalational agent & liberal titration of opioid
- Awaken & extubate in OR if lesion very small
- Often need manual bag ventilation during case as surgeon is attempting primary repair

- Constant communication with surgeon essential; needs to know effects of intraabdominal contents on SpO_2 & blood pressure
- Keep well paralyzed during case
- May need to defer primary repair & place silo for staged repair

PAIN MANAGEMENT

- Systemic: liberal titration of intraop fentanyl and postop if mechanically ventilated
- Regional: caudal epidural catheter can be used intraop; leave in place for postop analgesia

PACU/POSTOPERATIVE CONSIDERATIONS

- Abdominal compartment syndrome: hypoxemia, hypotension, oliguria
- Liberal paralysis if symptomatic
- Analgesia: continue epidural analgesia or opioid infusion

OPEN GLOBE INJURY REPAIR

PETE G. KOVATSIS, MD

CO-EXISTING DISEASES

- Intraocular press (IOP) increased by coughing, vomiting, crying, hypercarbia & hypoxia: can worsen clinical condition
- May be assoc with head & neck trauma
- Considered full stomach

PREOPERATIVE ASSESSMENT

- Studies: none
- Premed: midazolam prn, IV or PO
- Topical cream for IV placement
- Aspiration prophylaxis: metoclopramide, H_2 blockers, Na Bicitra
- Fentanyl (1–3 mcg/kg) can aid sedation & blunt induction response.

- NPO: std

PROCEDURAL CONSIDERATIONS
- Supine: bed rotated 90°
- Place IV preop.
- Monitors: std
- Oculocardiac reflex (OCR) possible: bradycardia: treat with atropine

ANESTHETIC PLAN
- RSI
- Minimize IOP increases.
- Although pre-O_2 important, avoid placing face mask on injured globe or struggling with child; both increase IOP.
- If child asleep without IV access, consider "steal" mask induction with cricoid pressure.
- Atropine 0.02 mg/kg for OCR & vagotonic reflexes assoc with sux & intubation.
- Prefer thiopental 4–6 mg/kg or thiopental + propofol to avoid painful injection that results in crying & struggling, leading to increased IOP
- NMB required
- Preference is sux 1.5–2 mg/kg for RSI: fast with short duration
- Sux controversial: increases IOP: up to 8 mmHg × 7 min
- This is less threatening to eye than suboptimal conditions or aspiration.
- Use with 1/10th intubating dose of nondepolarizing NMB before sux to minimize increased IOP
- ETT required
- Maintenance: balanced technique or TIVA
- Maintain muscle relaxation with NMB until perforation closed.
- Mild hypocarbia may decrease IOP.
- Empty stomach with OG tube after perforation closed.
- Minimize bucking & coughing at emergence.
- Deep extubation contraindicated if full stomach

■ Adjuvant tx: antiemetics to avoid vomiting & stress on sutures
■ May require arm restraints to avoid rubbing & injury

PAIN MANAGEMENT
■ Systemic: titrate fentanyl

PACU/POSTOPERATIVE CONSIDERATIONS
■ Systemic antibiotics
■ Analgesia: acetaminophen, and/or nonsteroidal often sufficient; otherwise titrate morphine

---

ORCHIDOPEXY (UNDESCENDED TESTICLE REPAIR)

PASQUALE DE NEGRI, MD

CO-EXISTING DISEASES
■ None

PREOPERATIVE ASSESSMENT
■ Studies: none
■ Premedication: if >1 yr, PO midazolam 0.5 mg/kg; max 15 mg
■ NPO: std

PROCEDURAL CONSIDERATIONS
■ Supine
■ IV fluids: LR; minimal bleeding & 3rd space loss
■ Monitors: std

ANESTHETIC PLAN
■ Inhalation induction with sevoflurane or IV induction with propofol or thiopental
■ NMB of choice to facilitate intubation or if using controlled ventilation
■ ETT or LMA
■ Maintenance: balanced technique: O_2, N_2O, volatile agent
■ Awaken & extubate in OR

PAIN MANAGEMENT

- Systemic: titrate intraop fentanyl or alfentanil or morphine 0.05 mg/kg
- Regional: caudal or hernia block

PACU/POSTOPERATIVE CONSIDERATIONS

- Analgesia: PR acetaminophen 40 mg/kg, then 20 mg/kg q6h
- PO codeine 0.5-1.0 mg/kg; max 30 mg alone or with acetaminophen

---

OTOPLASTY

ALAN JAY SCHWARTZ, MD AND SEMYON FISHKIN, MD

CO-EXISTING DISEASES

- Maxillary & mandibular bony abnormalities assoc with difficult intubation (uncommon)
- Syndromes (Treacher Collins, Goldenhar, Pierre Robin, Prader-Willi) possible, but most ear deformities not assoc with syndromes
- Assoc with renal anomalies (uncommon)
    - ➤ Assoc with cardiac abnormalities (uncommon)
    - ➤ Assoc with vertebral/cervical spine abnormalities (uncommon)

PREOPERATIVE ASSESSMENT

- Studies: usually none; ECHO, kidney ultrasound, neck imaging as needed
- Premed: if >1 yr, PO midazolam 0.5 mg/kg; max 10 mg
- NPO: std

PROCEDURAL CONSIDERATIONS

- Position: supine with OR table 90–180°
- Slight head-up position may reduce bleeding.

- Epinephrine diluted with saline or mixed with local anesthetic injected into surgical field
- IV fluids: LR
- Blood loss & 3rd space losses usually minimal
- Autogenous costal cartilage for reconstruction of external ear may be harvested from child's ribs (pneumothorax may occur when costal cartilage harvested) or iliac crest; will acutely increase child's anesthetic requirement
- Monitors: std
- Risks: ETT disconnection or displacement, epi or local anesthetic toxicity
- Calculate epi (max 10 mcg/kg; if halothane used, limit to 1 mcg/kg) & local anesthetic dose limits before injection & tell surgeon; dilution allows greater volume to be injected when surgical area extensive

ANESTHETIC PLAN
- Routine mask or IV induction with agents of choice if no airway distortion
- Oral RAE ETT in midline; anesthesia circuit follows longitudinal axis of pt
- Maintenance: balanced technique with agents & NMBs of choice
- Caution with halothane if surgeon infiltrates field with epi: may cause arrhythmias
- Awaken & extubate in OR

PAIN MANAGEMENT
- Systemic: titrate small doses of an opioid to produce a sedated emergence in pts who have dressings covering both ears & can't hear well
- Regional: local by surgeon

PACU/POSTOPERATIVE CONSIDERATIONS
- Hematoma formation, esp when epi wears off

- Analgesia: titrate opioid of choice
- CXR if costal cartilage harvested to rule out pneumothorax
- Possibility of atelectasis due to pain with chest movements
- Agitation when pts awaken with bilateral dressings covering external auditory openings & can't hear well

---

PATENT DUCTUS ARTERIOSUS (PDA) LIGATION

AISLING CONRAN, MD

CO-EXISTING DISEASES
- Incid 10% of CHD, inc risk if low birth weight
  - CHF: L to R shunt across ductus produces increased volume load on LV
  - Presentation: tachypnea, diaphoresis, freq URI, FTT
  - PE: continuous murmur (loudest at upper left sternal border), wide pulse pressure, 3–4+ pulses
- Associated intracardiac defects
- Prematurity
- Bronchopulmonary dysplasia (BPD)
- Intraventricular hemorrhage (IVH)

PREOPERATIVE ASSESSMENT
- Studies: hct
- Premed: none
- NPO: std

PROCEDURAL CONSIDERATIONS
- Position: lateral for L thoracotomy; supine for sternotomy, if assoc intracardiac defects also repaired
- IV fluids: need dextrose in prems
- Replace fluid deficits, blood loss & 3rd space loss with LR or NS.

- Monitors: std + pre- & postductal SpO_2, A-line R arm optional; BP will rise when ductus is ligated
- Thoracoscopic ligation is an option.
- Risks: injury to recurrent laryngeal nerve or thoracic duct; ligation of descending aorta, L pulmonary artery or carotid artery

ANESTHETIC PLAN

- Neonates & prems in CHF may not tolerate inhalation agents but will tolerate an opioid & NMB.
- Induction: IV opioids
- Maintenance: opioids (usually fentanyl) & NMB
- Emergence: extubation in OR likely with an older pt, but in prems prolonged postop weaning off ventilator is likely

PAIN MANAGEMENT

- Systemic: IV opioids
- Regional: in older child, consider caudal morphine

PACU/POSTOPERATIVE CONSIDERATIONS

- Analgesia: IV morphine 0.05 mg/kg prn; if intubated consider fentanyl infusion

---

PECTUS CARINATUM REPAIR

ORIGINALLY WRITTEN BY LORI STRICKER, MD
REVISED BY RONALD S. LITMAN, DO

CO-EXISTING DISEASES

- Marfan syndrome
- Congenital heart disease
- Mitral valve prolapse
- Pts typically asymptomatic; repair ideally after growth spurt

PREOPERATIVE ASSESSMENT

- Studies: hct, CXR, ECG
- Echo as indicated from H&P

- Premed: if >1 yr, PO midazolam 0.5 mg/kg; max 10 mg
- NPO: std

PROCEDURAL CONSIDERATIONS

- Supine
- Costal cartilage removed & position of sternum corrected
- IV fluids: LR for maintenance & replacement
- Minimal/moderate blood loss
- Monitors: std
- A-line if cardiopulmonary disease
- Risks: pneumothorax
- Sternal support rarely needed; transverse metal bar placed on ribs beneath sternum

ANESTHETIC PLAN

- Standard inhalational or IV induction
- NMBs may be used
- ETT required
- Maintenance: balanced technique of O_2, air & volatile agent
- Cautious use of N_2O due to risk of pneumothorax
- Awaken & extubate in OR unless CHD or high-dose opioid technique

PAIN MANAGEMENT

- Systemic: opioid of choice
- Regional: thoracolumbar epidural ideal for postop analgesia

PACU/POSTOPERATIVE CONSIDERATIONS

- Supplemental O_2 may be needed
- CXR to rule out pneumothorax or atelectasis
- Flail chest may occur with spontaneous ventilation.
- Atelectasis from manipulation of lung, splinting, hypoventilation
- Analgesia: consider morphine PCA, but continuation of epidural best

- Thoracic: 0.0625–0.125% bupivacaine + fentanyl 2–5 mcg/mL; run fentanyl at 1 mcg/kg/h
- Lumbar: 0.0625–0.125% bupivacaine + hydromorphone 0.01–0.02 mg/mL at 3 mcg/kg/h, or morphine 0.025–0.05 mg/mL at 8 mcg/kg/h
- IV ketorolac 0.5 mg/kg q6h

PECTUS EXCAVATUM REPAIR

ORIGINALLY WRITTEN BY LORI STRICKER, MD
REVISED BY DARRYL BERKOWITZ, MD

CO-EXISTING DISEASE

- Marfan's
- Congenital heart disease
- Mitral valve prolapse: up to 65%
- Scoliosis: up to 21%

PRE-OPERATIVE ASSESSMENT

- Cardiac: full assessment if assoc. CHD
- Severe cases: heart displaced to left and compressed, leading to RVOTO & arrhythmia, particularly with exercise & upright posture
- ECHO, ECG, CXR
- Pulmonary: Severe cases cause decreased lung volumes, forced expiratory flow & V:Q mismatch
- Labs: CBC, PT, PTT, T&S

PROCEDURAL CONSIDERATIONS

- Ravitch procedure: open procedure involving rib & costal cartilage resection, transverse sternal fracture with reconstruction involving sutures, adjacent ribs and metal plates posterior to sternal fracture line to bring sternum anterior
- Nuss procedure: less invasive, 2 small lateral incisions with pre-bent metal bar passed under ribs & sternum with curve

initially in wrong direction but flipped into correct curvature; bar remains for up to 2 years & removed

- No clear advantage between procedures; surgeon/institution dependent

ANESTHETIC PLAN

- Preop sedatives: careful if severe cardiorespiratory disease
- Monitors: std $\pm$ a-line if co-morbidities
- Induction: IV or volatile, 2 IV lines, oral ETT
- Maintenance: O_2/Air/Volatile (avoid N2O; potential pneumothorax)
- Position: supine, arms abducted
- Potential problems: arrhythmia during placement of Nuss bar, hemorrhage, pneumothorax, cardiac penetration
- Emergence: awaken & extubate in OR

PAIN MANAGEMENT

- Intraop: continuous epidural or IV opioid, NSAID

POST-OPERATIVE CONSIDERATIONS

- Pneumothorax/pleural effusion: up to 60%; usually resolve spontaneously
- Inadequate analgesia leads to atelectasis/ hypoventilation
- Flail chest

PELVIC OSTEOTOMY

RONALD S. LITMAN, DO

CO-EXISTING DISEASES

- Procedure indicated for correction of congenital hip dislocation
- Assoc with Down syndrome, arthrogryposis & chromosomal anomalies

PREOPERATIVE ASSESSMENT

- Studies: hct, T&S
- Premed: PO midazolam 0.5 mg/kg; max 10 mg
- NPO: std

PROCEDURAL CONSIDERATIONS

- Supine
- IV fluids: warmed LR
- 3rd space loss 3–5 mL/kg/h
- Potential for significant blood loss
- Monitors: std
- Risks: anemia, hypothermia

ANESTHETIC PLAN

- Inhalation or IV induction with agents of choice
- NMB helpful for intubation & surgical immobility
- ETT required
- Procedure usually lasts 2–4 h
- Maintenance: balanced technique: isoflurane, O_2, N_2O, NMB, opioid
- Plan for time at end of procedure for placement of spica cast.
- Awaken & extubate in OR

PAIN MANAGEMENT

- Systemic: if no regional, titrate intraop fentanyl or opioid of choice
- Regional: caudal catheter placed after induction: use intraop with 0.25% bupivacaine, 0.2% ropivacaine, 15% lidocaine, or 3% 2-chloroprocaine
- Epidural morphine 0.03–0.05 mg/kg
- Will need to tape catheter around spica cast at end of case

PACU/POSTOPERATIVE CONSIDERATIONS

- Analgesia: continue epidural local anesthetic of choice
- IV morphine 0.05 mg/kg prn

PERMANENT VASCULAR ACCESS (HICKMAN, BROVIAC, MEDIPORT CATHETER PLACEMENT)

MARIA M. ZESTOS, MD

CO-EXISTING DISEASES
- Chemotherapy, hemodialysis, prolonged antibiotic therapy & parenteral nutrition (TPN)
- Thoroughly evaluate comorbidity

PREOPERATIVE ASSESSMENT
- Studies: guided by comorbidity
- Cancer pts: hct, coags, date of last chemotx
- Renal failure patients: K, BUN, creatinine, date of last dialysis
- TPN patients: electrolytes
- Premed: IV or PO midazolam
- NPO: std

PROCEDURAL CONSIDERATIONS
- Supine, Trendelenburg, head turned to side, shoulder roll
- Radiolucent OR table
- Standard IV fluids
- Monitors: std
- Watch ECG for ectopy during wire & catheter placement
- Rare complications: cardiac tamponade, carotid artery injury, wire embolization
- Risks: arterial puncture, pneumothorax, vascular tear with hemothorax

ANESTHETIC PLAN
- Inhalational or IV induction
- All children should be intubated for maximum safety & surgical access.
- Maintenance: use of N_2O controversial because of risk of expansion of pneumothorax

- ■ Use balanced technique of O_2, air & volatile agent.
- ■ Awaken & extubate in OR

PAIN MANAGEMENT
- ■ Systemic: titrate fentanyl; avoid morphine & meperidine in pts with delayed renal clearance
- ■ Regional: local infiltration with 0.25% bupivacaine lessens postop pain

PACU/POSTOPERATIVE CONSIDERATIONS
- ■ Check CXR for line placement, hemothorax or pneumothorax
- ■ Analgesia: IV ketorolac 0.3 mg/kg and/or titrate fentanyl

---

POLLICIZATION

RONALD S. LITMAN, DO

CO-EXISTING DISEASES
- ■ Many different types of congenital syndromes: may include thrombocytopenia, Fanconi's anemia (pancytopenia), Holt-Oram syndrome (VSD or ASD)
- ■ Always look for other congenital defects.

PREOPERATIVE ASSESSMENT
- ■ Studies: none except if pt has known coexisting disease
- ■ May require SBE prophylaxis
- ■ Premed: if >1 yr, PO midazolam 0.5 mg/kg; max 15 mg
- ■ NPO: std

PROCEDURAL CONSIDERATIONS
- ■ Supine with OR table turned 90° to side of hand
- ■ Procedure involves transferring intact index finger to thumb location
- ■ IV fluids: LR; 3rd space loss minimal
- ■ Monitors: std
- ■ Risks: hyperthermia from overuse of warming devices

■ Tourniquet usually used

ANESTHETIC PLAN

■ Inhalation induction with sevo or halothane or IV induction with agent of choice
■ NMB of choice may be used to facilitate intubation.
■ ETT required
■ Maintenance: balanced technique: N_2O, O_2 & volatile agent
■ Awaken & extubate in OR

PAIN MANAGEMENT

■ Systemic: titrate intraop fentanyl
■ Regional: not usually performed because of concern of masking compartment syndrome when cast placed on upper extremity

PACU/POSTOPERATIVE CONSIDERATIONS

■ Analgesia: PO acetaminophen 10–15 mg q6h, ibuprofen 10 mg/kg q6h, codeine 1 mg/kg (max 30 mg) q6h

---

POSTERIOR SPINAL FUSION

CHERYL K. GOODEN, MD, FAAP

CO-EXISTING DISEASES

■ Neuromuscular disorders such as osteogenesis imperfecta, Marfan's, Ehlers-Danlos, neurofibromatosis, cerebral palsy, muscular dystrophy, poliomyelitis, mucopolysaccharidosis

PREOPERATIVE ASSESSMENT

■ Determine etiology & degree of curvature: Cobb's angle $>65°$ assoc with restrictive lung disease
■ Assess CV impairment
■ Mitral valve prolapse in 25% of pts with scoliosis
■ Studies: hct, T&C

- PFTs & ABG if significant restrictive disease; if VC <30% predicted, may need postop ventilation
- ECG and/or echo if pulmonary htn, RVH or cor pulmonale suspected
- If wake-up test planned then discuss with pt
- Premed: PO midazolam 0.5 mg/kg; max 20 mg
- NPO: std

PROCEDURAL CONSIDERATIONS
- Prone
- IV fluids: warmed LR or any balanced salt solution
- 3rd space loss 8–10 mL/kg/h
- 2 large-bore IVs or 1 + central line
- Significant blood loss common
- Monitors: std + A-line + CVP + urinary catheter
- If SSEPs and/or MEPs used, need to keep volatile agent <0.2% & rely mainly on N_2O/narcotic technique + hypotensive agent for BP control
- Risks: hypothermia, hypotension, pneumothorax, nerve injury (from improper positioning), visual loss (secondary to ischemic optic neuropathy or retinal artery occlusion)

ANESTHETIC PLAN
- Inhalation or IV induction
- NMB of choice
- Maintenance: balanced technique: N_2O, O_2, inhalation agent, NMB, opioid (infusion preferred with SSEPs monitoring)
- Adjuvant tx: alternatives to homologous blood transfusion include advanced donation of autologous blood, acute normovolemic hemodilution & cell saver
- Choices for hypotensive technique include beta-blockers (labetalol, esmolol), nitroprusside & nicardipine
- Do not use both hemodilution & hypotension together: safety unproven
- Awaken & extubate in OR when possible

PAIN MANAGEMENT

- Systemic: fentanyl or other opioid OK: consider intraop infusion
- Spinal morphine: 0.005 mg/kg can be injected after induction or under direct vision by surgeon; duration of analgesia 12–18 h

PACU/POSTOPERATIVE CONSIDERATIONS

- PCA opioids immed postop or when intrathecal morphine wears off
- Cognitively impaired pts will require continuous infusion of morphine or fentanyl.
- Wound bleeding expected: usually drop hct by 2–3%
- Expect significant facial edema, resolves by 24 h

POSTERIOR URETHRAL VALVE REPAIR

PASQUALE DE NEGRI, MD

CO-EXISTING DISEASES

- Severe cases: renal failure, respiratory distress, sepsis, fluid & electrolyte abnormalities

PREOPERATIVE ASSESSMENT

- Studies: none unless indicated for renal eval
- Premed: if >1 yr, PO midazolam 0.5 mg/kg; max 15 mg
- NPO: std

PROCEDURAL CONSIDERATIONS

- Supine
- IV fluids: LR at maintenance
- Minimal bleeding or 3rd space loss
- Monitors: std

ANESTHETIC PLAN
- Inhalation induction with sevoflurane or IV induction with propofol or thiopental
- NMB of choice to facilitate intubation or if using controlled ventilation
- ETT or LMA
- Maintenance: balanced technique: O_2, N_2O, volatile agent
- Awaken & extubate in OR

PAIN MANAGEMENT
- Systemic: titrate intraop fentanyl or alfentanil
- Regional: caudal or penile block (see Circumcision chapter)

PACU/POSTOPERATIVE CONSIDERATIONS
- Analgesia: PR acetaminophen 40 mg/kg, then 20 mg/kg q6h
- PO codeine 0.5–1.0 mg/kg, max 30 mg alone or with acetaminophen

---

PULL-THROUGHS FOR HIRSCHSPRUNG'S DISEASE

CHRISTIAN SEEFELDER, MD

CO-EXISTING DISEASES
- Bowel obstruction
- 4–5% CHD
- 4–5% trisomy 21

PREOPERATIVE ASSESSMENT
- Studies: neonate: hct, blood glucose, T&S
- Premed: if >1 yr, PO midazolam 0.5 mg/kg; max 15 mg
- NPO: std, may have NGT, may have had bowel prep

PROCEDURAL CONSIDERATIONS
- Initial suction biopsy in the NICU without anesthesia
- Sick/unstable: neonatal colostomy, pull-through/colostomy closure in infancy

- Healthy: neonatal primary pull-through; may use laparoscopy
- Supine
- Pt at end of bed for pull-through, possibly across table: difficult access
- Intermittently Trendelenburg, lithotomy
- Gas insuff causes CV (hypotension) & resp (decreased compliance, hypercapnia) changes
- IV fluids: maintenance 4 mL/kg/h, neonates <1 wk: D10W, <3 mo D5 0.2–0.45% NS, >3 mo LR
- Consider blood sugar checks intraop
- Additional/3rd space loss LR, >=10 mL/kg/h for laparotomy
- Blood loss minimal
- Colloid (albumin 5%) and blood avail if neonate
- Monitors: std; A-line in neonates if laparoscopic or long procedure
- Risks: CV & resp depression if laparoscopy (intraabdominal pressure ideally <6 mmHg)
- Hypothermia: forced warm air & fluid warmers

ANESTHETIC PLAN

- IV or inhalation OK
- Nondepolarizing NMB
- Orotracheal intubation, OG/NG tube
- Vomiting/bowel obstruction: IV RSI: sux or roc
- Maintenance: balanced
- Awaken & extubate in OR

PAIN MANAGEMENT

- Systemic: without regional: fentanyl 1–2 mcg/kg or morphine 0.05–0.1 mg/kg
- Epidural: singledose caudal: 0.125–0.25% bupivacaine, max 1 mL/kg, consider redosing after long cases
- Catheter: lumbar or caudal (might be in surgical prep field)
- Or: infiltration of surgical site: bupivacaine 0.25%, up to 1 mL/kg

PACU/POSTOPERATIVE CONSIDERATIONS
- Analgesia: cont epidural infusion: 0.05–0.1% bupivacaine ± low-dose fentanyl or 1.5% chloroprocaine, 0.2–0.3 mL/kg
- Systemic: morphine: neonates: 0.025–0.05 mg/kg IV q4h prn; infants & children: 0.05–0.1 mg/kg IV q2h prn
- Acetaminophen: 15 mg/kg PO q4h, q6h in neonates
- NSAIDs: (except neonates and young infants)
  - ibuprofen 5–10 mg/kg PO q8h
  - ketorolac 0.25 mg/kg IV q8h
- Follow neonates & young infants receiving systemic/epidural narcotics closely with apnea/ECG/SpO_2 monitor/consider NICU

PULMONARY SEQUESTRATION

RONALD S. LITMAN, DO

CO-EXISTING DISEASES
- Recurrent pneumonia, chronic cough
- Rare: other congenital anomalies

PREOPERATIVE ASSESSMENT
- Studies: none
- Premed: if > 1 yr, PO midazolam 0.5 mg/kg; max 10 mg
- NPO: std

PROCEDURAL CONSIDERATIONS
- Sequestration is a nonfunctional mass of lung tissue supplied by anomalous systemic arteries.
- Arterial supply arises from aorta; venous drainage usually through pulmonary veins
- Does not usually become inflated with positive-pressure ventilation
- Surgeon may require OLV (see VATS chapter for detailed mgmt)

- Position: lat decub
- IV fluids: LR, 3rd space loss 5–8 mL/kg/h
- Monitors: std
- Risks: hypoxemia during OLV

ANESTHETIC PLAN
- Induction: IV or inhalational of choice
- Maintenance: balanced technique with O_2, air & volatile agent
- Avoid N_2O
- Awaken & extubate in OR

PAIN MANAGEMENT
- Systemic: titrate fentanyl or opioid of choice
- Regional: thoracic epidural – can be placed via lumbar or caudal approach

PACU/POSTOPERATIVE CONSIDERATIONS
- Analgesia: continue epidural if present
- IV morphine 0.05–0.1 mg/kg prn
- IV ketorolac 0.5 mg/kg q6h
- CXR to R/O pneumothorax

PYLOROMYOTOMY

ORIGINALLY WRITTEN BY FANNIE SCHAPIRO, MD
REVISED BY RONALD S. LITMAN, DO

CO-EXISTING DISEASES
- 2% will develop jaundice from glucuronyl-transferase deficiency – resolves after surgery
- Delayed gastric emptying, gastric dilatation, regurgitation & nonbilious projectile vomiting
- Persistent vomiting leads to dehydration, wt loss, anemia, electrolyte imbalance & alkalosis.

- Typical derangement is hypochloremic, hypokalemic metabolic alkalosis.

PREOPERATIVE ASSESSMENT
- Studies: H/H, lytes
- Must have adequate fluid resuscitation & normal lytes before surgery
- Never a surgical emergency
- Premed: none
- NPO at time of dx

PROCEDURAL CONSIDERATIONS
- Supine
- IV fluids: LR, 3rd space loss usually 1–2 mL/kg/h
- D5LR or NS for maintenance
- Fluids should be warmed
- Minimal blood loss
- Monitors: std
- Risks: aspiration of gastric contents during induction, postop apnea

ANESTHETIC PLAN
- Before induction: empty stomach with 10 or 12F suction catheter
- O_2 by mask & IV atropine 0.02 mg/kg; min dose 0.15 mg
- Choices: awake intubation or RSI with cricoid pressure
- Induction agents: pentothal or propofol
- NMB for intubation: sux or roc
- Hypoxemia from apnea during RSI common; must usually ventilate before intubation
- Maintenance: N_2O, O_2 & volatile agent
- Maintain SpO_2 95–100%
- Any short- or intermed-acting NMB
- Emergence: reverse NMB

- Awaken & extubate in OR
- Delayed awakening common

PAIN MANAGEMENT
- Opioids generally avoided
- Remifentanil OK
- Regional: local infiltration with 0.25% bupivacaine by surgeon before closure

PACU/POSTOPERATIVE CONSIDERATIONS
- Analgesia: acetaminophen usually sufficient
- Two main risks are central apnea & reactive hypoglycemia.
- Supplemental O_2 in PACU
- Continue IV glucose solution until adequate PO intake
- Pulse ox/apnea monitor for first 12–24 h

RADIOTHERAPY

ORIGINALLY WRITTEN BY ABBOY MOHAN, MD
REVISED BY RONALD S. LITMAN, DO

CO-EXISTING DISEASES
- Brain tumors
- Assoc neuro problems: ICP, seizures, cranial nerve involvement
- Bone marrow depression or cardiotoxicity from chemotx

PREOPERATIVE ASSESSMENT
- Studies: none
- Premed: usually none
- NPO: std; make sure treatments are scheduled early in AM so pt doesn't need to be NPO for very long
- If two treatments per day, allow liberal clears up to 2 hours before afternoon tx

PROCEDURAL CONSIDERATIONS

- Position: supine or prone
- Absolute immobility needed
- Often use constricting face mask that interferes with airway
- Procedure lasts 4–15 min: 1 or 2 sessions a day.
- Tx can last up to 6 weeks.
- Gamma knife: stereotactic radiotx for vascular malformation or brain tumor involves placement of head frame, CT & MRI
- Pts may need sedation while waiting for computation of orientation of radiation.
- IV fluids: any at maintenance
- Monitors: remote-controlled TV camera used to observe monitors; standard monitors & nasal cannula with capnograph
- Risks: airway obstruction, pt movement during tx

ANESTHETIC PLAN

- Pts usually have existing long-term indwelling IV access; if not consider placement of PICC line at 1st tx.
- Induction: propofol 2–3 mg/kg IV slowly while maintaining spont ventilation
- Alternatives: ketamine or inhalation agents
- Intubation best avoided
- Maintenance: propofol 200–300 mcg/kg/min
- Pts usually go home shortly after emergence
- Adjuvant tx: consider PO or IV anticholinergic agents for excessive drooling (eg, glycopyrrolate 0.01 mg/kg/IV)

PAIN MANAGEMENT

- None required

PACU/POSTOPERATIVE CONSIDERATIONS

- None

RETROPHARYNGEAL ABSCESS

RONALD S. LITMAN, DO

CO-EXISTING DISEASES
- Usually none

PREOPERATIVE ASSESSMENT
- Studies: none
- Premed: PO midazolam 0.5 mg/kg only if upper airway obstruction absent
- NPO: often full stomach
- Obtain IV access preop
- Examine radiologic studies to assess severity of airway obstruction.

PROCEDURAL CONSIDERATIONS
- Supine
- Table turned; pt in tonsil position
- IV fluids: any OK; 3rd space loss minimal
- Monitors: std
- Risks: hypoxemia from upper airway obstruction

ANESTHETIC PLAN
- Keep spontaneous ventilation until proven that positive-pressure ventilation successful
- Inhalation with sevo & 100% O_2 or slow IV induction with pentothal or propofol
- When pt deeply sedated, gently try to assist ventilation: if success, administer NMB and continue with conventional induction & intubation
- If air entry unsuccessful with positive pressure, keep breathing spontaneously & prepare for deep intubation or (rare) tracheostomy

- Maintenance: balanced technique: volatile agent, O_2, N_2O & opioid
- Awaken & extubate in OR
- Rarely keep ventilated postop
- Dexamethasone 0.5 mg/kg, max 10 mg, to decrease airway swelling

PAIN MANAGEMENT
- Systemic: titrate small amt of intraop fentanyl
- Regional: none

PACU/POSTOPERATIVE CONSIDERATIONS
- Airway obstruction

SLIPPED CAPITAL FEMORAL EPIPHYSIS (SCFE) REPAIR

RONALD S. LITMAN, DO

CO-EXISTING DISEASES
- Usually obese adolescents
- Rare: underlying hypothyroidism or renal osteodystrophy

PREOPERATIVE ASSESSMENT
- Studies: hct, lytes, creat, T&S
- Premed: IV/PO midazolam, 0.5 mg/kg; max 10 mg
- NPO: std

PROCEDURAL CONSIDERATIONS
- Placement of pin through acetabulum & femoral head
- Supine or lateral decub
- IV fluids: warmed LR
- 3rd space loss 3-6 mL/kg/h
- Monitors: std
- Risks: positioning injuries if pt obese

ANESTHETIC PLAN
- IV or inhalation induction & intubation with agents of choice
- Modified RSI if obese
- Maintenance: balanced technique: O_2, N_2O, isoflurane, NMB, opioid
- Awaken & extubate in OR

PAIN MANAGEMENT
- Systemic: titrate intraop fentanyl or opioid of choice
- Regional: one-shot caudal injection of 0.25% bupivacaine 0.5 mL/kg with epi & morphine 0.03 mg/kg; catheter for postop pain usually unnecessary

PACU/POSTOPERATIVE CONSIDERATIONS
- Analgesia: IV morphine 0.05 mg/kg prn; PO oxycodone 0.1 mg/kg q4-6h prn

---

SPLENECTOMY

PETE G. KOVATSIS, MD

CO-EXISTING DISEASES
- ITP, anemias (hereditary spherocytosis, thalassemia), myelo- or lymphoproliferative disorders, trauma, hypersplenism
- Myocardial depression due to XRT or chemotherapy (CRX)
- Respiratory compromise secondary to splenomegaly, XRT or CRX
- Cytopenias
- Neurologic, renal, hepatic function affected by CRX

PREOPERATIVE ASSESSMENT
- Studies: CBC, coags, T&C
- Premed: midazolam, IV or PO

- Stress steroids as needed
- NPO: std

PROCEDURAL CONSIDERATIONS
- Position: supine or semilateral
- IV fluids: warmed LR; 3rd space loss 10–15 mL/kg/h
- Blood loss <5% of blood volume, but prepare for major bleeding
- Monitors: std
- Avoid hypothermia: forced warm air blanket & fluid warmer
- Increased chance of blood loss with splenorrhaphy or subtotal splenectomy

ANESTHETIC PLAN
- Mask or IV induction of choice
- Consider RSI if splenomegaly or hepatosplenomegaly impinges on gastroesophageal function
- NMB required: no preferred agent
- ETT required
- Maintenance: balanced technique
- Epidural anesthesia beneficial for open if not coagulopathic
- Avoid N_2O to prevent bowel distention
- Awake extubation

PAIN MANAGEMENT
- Systemic: titrate opioids
- Regional: if epidural present, 0.25% bupivacaine intraop

PACU/POSTOPERATIVE CONSIDERATIONS
- Complications: bleeding, respiratory compromise, sepsis (overwhelming post-splenectomy infection) or subphrenic abscess
- Thrombocytosis & DVT
- Pancreatitis or pancreatic fistula
- Analgesia: prefer continuous epidural infusions but PCA, NCA, or prn IV morphine OK

STRABISMUS REPAIR

ORIGINALLY WRITTEN BY PEDRO P. VANZILLOTTA, MD
REVISED BY RONALD S. LITMAN, DO

CO-EXISTING DISEASES
■ CNS: cerebral palsy, hydrocephalus, meningomyelocele
■ Myopathies
■ Wide variety of congenital & chromosomal syndromes

PREOPERATIVE ASSESSMENT
■ Studies: none
■ Premed: midazolam
■ NPO: std

PROCEDURAL CONSIDERATIONS
■ Supine; OR table turned 90°
■ If unilateral repair, unprepped eye must have upper lid taped shut
■ IV fluids: LR at maintenance
■ Monitors: std
■ Risks: manipulation of extraocular muscles, mainly medial rectus, may induce OCR, resulting in bradycardia or, less frequently, other cardiac dysrhythmias: junctional rhythm, AV block, PVCs, V-tach & asystole

ANESTHETIC PLAN
■ Inhalation or IV induction, no preferred agent
■ ETT or LMA required and taped securely; some prefer oral RAE
■ NMBs may be used to facilitate intubation or at surgeon's request to remove any interference with forced duction testing.
■ Maintenance: sevo or desflurane
■ Depth of anesthesia should be at a level to maintain the eyes in the straight-ahead position.

- Light anesthesia & hypercarbia augment incidence & severity of OCR.
- Awaken & extubate in OR
- Adjuvant tx: OCR treatment: slow & gentle muscle traction usually leads to reflex fatigue, otherwise atropine 0.02 mg/kg or glycopyrrolate 0.01 mg/kg to treat worrisome or repeated bradycardia

PAIN MANAGEMENT
- Topical: Tetracaine eye drops
- Systemic: PR acetaminophen 30–40 mg/kg + IV ketorolac 0.3–0.5 mg/kg

PACU/POSTOPERATIVE CONSIDERATIONS
- Analgesia: mild systemic analgesics usually sufficient
- More intense pain should prompt reexamination.
- IV ondansetron 0.05 mg/kg, dimenhydrinate 0.3–0.5 mg/kg or metoclopramide 0.15 mg/kg may be used after induction.
- Recommend delayed feeding & avoid early ambulation.
- Restlessness due to eye irritation, blurred vision or eye occlusion

---

SYNDACTYLY REPAIR

RONALD S. LITMAN, DO

CO-EXISTING DISEASES
- Many different types of congenital syndromes: may include heart defects and difficult intubation (Apert's syndrome)
- Always look for other congenital defects.

PREOPERATIVE ASSESSMENT
- Studies: none except if pt has known coexisting disease
- May require SBE prophylaxis if congenital heart disease
- Premed: if >1 yr, PO midazolam 0.5 mg/kg; max 10 mg
- NPO: std

PROCEDURAL CONSIDERATIONS

- Supine with OR table turned 90° to side of limb involved
- Procedure involves surgical excision of web between fingers or toes.
- IV fluids: LR; 3rd space loss minimal
- Monitors: std
- Risks: hyperthermia from overuse of warming devices
- Tourniquet usually used.

ANESTHETIC PLAN

- Inhalation induction with sevoflurane or IV induction with agent of choice
- NMB of choice may be used to facilitate intubation
- ETT or LMA
- Maintenance: balanced technique with N_2O, O_2 & volatile agent
- Awaken & extubate in OR

PAIN MANAGEMENT

- Systemic: titrate intraop fentanyl
- Regional: one-shot axillary block or caudal injection of local anesthetic; use 0.25–0.5 mL/kg 0.25% bupivacaine
- Digital blocks also OK

PACU/POSTOPERATIVE CONSIDERATIONS

- Analgesia choices: IV ketorolac 0.5 mg/kg; acetaminophen 40 mg/kg PR in OR, then 20 mg/kg q6h; ibuprofen 10 mg/kg q6h
- Opioids usually not necessary

TESTICULAR TORSION REPAIR

PASQUALE DE NEGRI, MD

CO-EXISTING DISEASES

- None

PREOPERATIVE ASSESSMENT
- Studies: none
- Premed: if >1 yr, PO midazolam 0.5 mg/kg; max 15 mg
- NPO: full stomach since usually surgical emergency

PROCEDURAL CONSIDERATIONS
- Supine
- IV fluids: LR at maintenance
- Minimal bleeding or 3rd space loss
- Monitors: std

ANESTHETIC PLAN
- RSI: propofol or thiopental; NMB with sux or roc
- Maintenance: balanced technique: O_2, N_2O, volatile agent
- Awaken & extubate in OR

PAIN MANAGEMENT
- Systemic: titrate intraop fentanyl or alfentanil
- Regional: hernia block or local by surgeon

PACU/POSTOPERATIVE CONSIDERATIONS
- Analgesia: PR acetaminophen 40 mg/kg, then 20 mg/kg q6h
- PO codeine 0.5–1.0 mg/kg; max 30 mg alone or with acetaminophen

---

TETRALOGY OF FALLOT REPAIR

SCOTT WALKER, MD

CO-EXISTING DISEASES
- VSD, RV outflow tract (RVOT) obstruction, RVH, pulmonary stenosis or atresia, double-outlet RV, aortopulmonary collaterals
- Cyanotic (tet) spells: provoked by hypercontractility, inc PVR, or dec SVR assoc with agitation or administration of vasodilators

- Tx: O_2, volume, phenylephrine 1–2 mcg/kg, propranolol 150 mcg/kg, morphine 25–50 mcg/kg
- Hip flexion and/or abdominal compression (if chest open, aortic compression)
- High-pressure ventilation may exacerbate tet spell by inc PVR.

PREOPERATIVE ASSESSMENT
- Studies: echo, cardiac cath data, room air SpO_2
- Premed: if >1 yr, PO midazolam 0.5 mg/kg; max 15 mg
- NPO: std

PROCEDURAL CONSIDERATIONS
- Palliative repair: BT shunt (systemic to PA)
- Definitive repair: VSD patch, RVOT muscle resection & possibly pulmonary transannular patch ± "monocusp" pulmonary homograft valve
- May involve R ventriculotomy on CPB
- Position: definitive repair: supine; BT shunt: lateral decub
- IV fluids: maintain normovolemia with volume; albumin/crystalloid readily available to treat tet spell
- Monitors: std + A-line ± CVP
- Risks: tet spell during induction & emergence but may occur intraop, during surgical stimulation or manipulation of pulmonary vessels

ANESTHETIC PLAN
- Weigh potential for systemic vasodilation during inhalation induction vs. hypercontractility assoc with agitation during awake IV insertion.
- Gradual sevo induction usually well tolerated even in cyanotic pts.
- Ketamine, 1–2 mg/kg, also OK
- Maintenance (BT shunt): remifentanil provides stable technique while preserving option for postop extubation
- Low-dose volatile agent or benzo for amnesia

- Maintenance (definitive repair): any opioid + volatile agent and/or benzo
- Emergence: awaken & extubate in OR after BT shunt if CXR OK, normothermia & good analgesia
- After definitive repair continue opioids & intubation.

PAIN MANAGEMENT
- Systemic: for BT shunt: remifentanil, 0.2–1.0 mcg/kg/min; for definitive repair: liberal doses of any opioid titrated to CV response
- Regional: intercostal nerve block or local by surgeon
- Caudal epidural: preservative-free morphine 50–100 mcg/kg, in NS-0.5 mL/kg total volume
- Continuous wound infiltration: elastomeric local anesthetic infusion system

PACU/POSTOPERATIVE CONSIDERATIONS
- Arrhythmias, hypotension, ventilatory dependence
- Analgesia: morphine or meperidine prn or PCA

THYROGLOSSAL DUCT CYST

ALAN JAY SCHWARTZ, MD

CO-EXISTING DISEASES
- Very rare: malignant thyroid degeneration

PREOPERATIVE ASSESSMENT
- Airway eval: distortion of airway from lingual thyroid very rare
- Studies: thyroid function if symptomatic
- Premed: if >1 yr, PO midazolam 0.5 mg/kg; max 10 mg
- NPO: std

PROCEDURAL CONSIDERATIONS
- Neck extended for transverse midline incision

- Oral cavity accessible to anesthesiologist: may be asked to depress base of the tongue to move cyst to facilitate surgical ID of proximal lingual attachment
- Slight head-up position may reduce bleeding.
- IV fluids: LR
- Blood loss and 3rd space replacement minimal
- Monitors: std
- Risks: surgical misadventure into vascular or airway structures

ANESTHETIC PLAN

- Routine mask or IV induction with agents of choice in child without airway distortion
- Intubation: oral ETT
- Nasal RAE OK also
- Maintenance: balanced with agents of choice
- Awaken & extubate in OR

PAIN MANAGEMENT

- Systemic: titrate opioid of choice
- Regional: local by surgeon

PACU/POSTOPERATIVE CONSIDERATIONS

- Vigilance for unsuspected hematoma formation (extremely rare) potentially compressing vascular and/or airway structures in neck
- Analgesia: titrate oral or IV opioid of choice

TONSILLAR ABSCESS DRAINAGE

MARIA M. ZESTOS, MD

CO-EXISTING DISEASES

- Acute pharyngotonsillitis
- Trismus, torticollis & inflammation: poss difficult intubation

PREOPERATIVE ASSESSMENT
- Studies: none
- Premed: midazolam; avoid if airway obstruction evident
- NPO: std

PROCEDURAL CONSIDERATIONS
- Supine, Trendelenburg in case abscess ruptures
- IV fluids: LR or NS; check volume status
- High fever, severe throat pain & difficulty swallowing may result in dehydration.
- Monitors: std
- Risks: spontaneous rupture of abscess may occur & fill pharynx with pus

ANESTHETIC PLAN
- Inhalation induction with spontaneous ventilation
- Avoid NMB: airway obstruction may occur
- May administer NMB if able to ventilate easily with positive pressure
- Consider lidocaine 1 mg/kg IV if not using NMB.
- Intubate trachea when pt deeply anesthetized if no NMB
- Use caution to avoid rupture of abscess during laryngoscopy.
- Oral RAE ETT
- Maintenance: balanced technique: O_2, N_2O & volatile agent
- Awaken & extubate in OR: fully awake with head turned to affected side

PAIN MANAGEMENT
- Systemic: titrate small doses of opioids (draining abscess produces immediate relief)

PACU/POSTOPERATIVE CONSIDERATIONS
- Post-extubation obstruction may occur due to pharyngeal swelling.
- Analgesia: IV ketorolac 0.3 mg/kg or titrate small doses of opioids

TONSILLECTOMY & ADENOIDECTOMY

FRANCINE S. YUDKOWITZ, MD, FAAP

CO-EXISTING DISEASES
- Sleep apnea: chronic hypoxemia may lead to polycythemia, pulmonary hypertension & cor pulmonale

PREOPERATIVE ASSESSMENT
- Studies: hct, CXR, ECG if suspect cardiopulmonary disease
- Coags if history of bleeding
- Premed: PO midazolam 0.5 mg/kg; max 15 mg
- Reduce midazolam dose if preexisting airway obstruction.
- Beware: pts may obstruct after sedatives
- NPO: std

PROCEDURAL CONSIDERATIONS
- Supine, neck extended
- OR table turned 90°
- IV fluids: isotonic crystalloid to replace deficit & blood loss
- Monitors: std
- Risks: sharing airway with surgeon, ETT kinking/dislodging (watch PIPs), arrhythmias, blood loss

ANESTHETIC PLAN
- Inhalation or IV induction
- Intubation with oral RAE or flexible LMA
- NMB may be used for intubation
- Maintenance: balanced technique or TIVA
- NMB not necessary
- Emergence: surgeon suctions pharynx (stomach optional) before extubation
- Extubation usually wide-awake, in lateral position with head slightly down

- Some prefer deep extubation but higher risk of postop laryngospasm
- Adjuvant tx: antiemetic, dexamethasone

PAIN MANAGEMENT
- Local anesthetic infiltration by surgeon to surgical site, but some evidence that this increases bleeding
- PR acetaminophen 40 mg/kg
- Intraop opioid of choice

PACU/POSTOPERATIVE CONSIDERATIONS
- Airway obstruction
- Some pts with sleep apnea need respiratory monitoring overnight.
- Emesis
- Postop bleed may go undetected & difficult to quantify.
- Inadequate PO intake

TOTAL ANOMALOUS PULMONARY VENOUS RETURN (TAPVR) REPAIR

AISLING CONRAN, MD

CO-EXISTING DISEASES
- 4 types: supracardiac (37–45%) drain into SVC, left SVC or innominate; cardiac (13–23%) drain into RA or coronary sinus; infracardiac (21–46%) drain below diaphragm; mixed connections (4–11%) 1% of all CHD (TAPVR & PAPVR)
- All, except cardiac, can obstruct, leading to inc PVR.
- Assoc cardiac defects or pulmonary sequestration
- L to R shunt of TAPVR is offset by R to L shunt by ASD or PFO.
- If R to L shunt restrictive, RV failure may occur from volume overload. LA blood flow is limited, dec CO, inc RAP & PAP

- If ASD is large (nonrestrictive) then pulmonary blood flow determined by ratio of PVR to SVR
- Clinical presentation depends on degree of obstruction of pulmonary veins; inc obstruction leads to inc cyanosis.
- Tachypnea, cyanosis, dec CO, dec systemic perfusion, right-sided CHF (large liver)

PREOPERATIVE ASSESSMENT
- Studies: hct, ABG
- Premed: none
- NPO: std

PROCEDURAL CONSIDERATIONS
- Supine
- IV fluid: dextrose in maintenance
- Monitors: std + A-line, LA, RA & PA lines by surgeon
- TEE: verify preop diagnosis & evaluate undiagnosed defects, adequacy of repair & ventricular fn
- Deep hypothermic circ arrest

ANESTHETIC PLAN
- Induction: if IV titrate opioids + NMB
- Alt: IM ketamine 2 mg/kg; mask induction not well tolerated
- If partial (PAPVR), inhalation induction usually tolerated
- Maintenance: opioids & NMB
- Frequent ABGs
- Off CPB: may require inotrope & vasodilator
- If PVR raised: physiologic goals include hypocarbia, oxygenation & alkalosis
- Pulmonary vasodilators include inhaled NO, nitroglycerin & nitroprusside.
- Maintain low LA pressure to prevent fluid overload: RA < 10–12

- Pacemaker may be needed (AV node may be damaged during repair).
- Adjuvant tx: ECMO

PAIN MANAGEMENT
- Titrate opioids

PACU/POSTOPERATIVE CONSIDERATIONS
- Inc PVR; pulmonary venous obstruction; RV failure; altered L heart hemodynamics after repair; arrhythmias: SVT (5–20%) in pts with cardiac APVR
- Sources of dec SpO_2: ASD, coronary sinus draining into LA; pulmonary edema; dec CO
- If obstructed veins preop, expect vent support for several days.
- Analgesia: fentanyl infusion for intubated pts Operative mortality is high. Inc if age <1 mo, pulm veins obstructed preop, dec LV fn, poor condition, other cardiac anomalies.

TRACHEAL RECONSTRUCTION

RICHARD ROWE, MD, MPH

CO-EXISTING DISEASES
- If trach in situ, symptoms of chronic bronchitis: airway secretions, atelectasis, bronchospasm, V/Q mismatch
- If hx of prematurity & BPD: often require bronchodilator tx

PREOPERATIVE ASSESSMENT
- Studies: CBC, lytes, T&C
- Premed: if >1 yr, PO midazolam 0.5 mg/kg; max 15 mg

PROCEDURAL CONSIDERATIONS
- Monitors: std + A-line, CVP, Foley
- Bilateral axillary stethoscopes
- Monitor ABG, glucose, lytes, hct

- IV fluids: LR; deficit + 3rd space: 5 mL/kg/h + maint D5$\frac{1}{2}$NS
- Major risk: hypoventilation or hypoxemia during reconstruction
- After prep, sterile cuffed ETT replaces trach tube.
- ETT is marked with suture at skin level to remind surgeons not to move ETT too far in or out.
- If no trach, consider ventilating through rigid bronch or small ETT.
- When surgeon has opened trachea, advance sterile ETT into proximal trachea, confirm breath sounds & mark ETT again.
- After posterior graft in place, advance ETT through glottis & have surgeon advance into trachea, securely tape into place.

ANESTHETIC PLAN
- Inhalation induction via trach or mask
- If no trach & critical subglottic stenosis, have plan available to ventilate pt before administration of NMB.
- Maintenance: balanced technique with air, O_2, volatile agent, opioid
- Most peds pts remain intubated for 7 days postop; adults usually extubated in OR
- Do not allow pt to cough: use IV opioids and/or lidocaine at extubation.
- If tracheal stenosis extends to carina or below, CPB may be required during placement of tracheal grafts if control of ventilation in distal airway impossible.

PAIN MANAGEMENT
- Systemic: titrate opioid to hemodynamics

PACU/POSTOPERATIVE CONSIDERATIONS
- Peds pt: keep paralyzed, do not allow neck to move, careful suctioning of ETT, eval for extubation in 7 days
- Adults: avoid coughing

TRACHEOESOPHAGEAL FISTULA & ESOPHAGEAL ATRESIA REPAIR

FRANKLYN P. CLADIS, MD

CO-EXISTING DISEASES
- Vertebral anomalies
- Anorectal/intestinal anomalies & atresia
- Cardiac defects
- Renal & radial anomalies
- Prematurity: RDS

PREOPERATIVE ASSESSMENT
- Studies: Hgb, glucose, echocardiography, renal ultrasound, radiographic exam of vertebrae
- Premedication: none
- Pts are NPO at time of dx; should have orogastric tube to drain esophageal pouch

PROCEDURAL CONSIDERATIONS
- Position: gastrostomy performed supine & head up; surgical repair in left lateral decub for right thoracotomy
- Surgery: ligation of TEF & anastomosis of atretic esophagus; if gap between esophageal segments too large for primary anastomosis, staged repair performed; usually colonic interposition
- IV fluids: D10W +0.2% normal saline for maintenance; LR or albumin for volume replacement
- Monitor blood glucose hourly
- Additional IV recommended
- 3rd space loss > 15 mL/kg/h
- Monitors: standard ASA monitors; A-line optional

- Esophageal stethoscope on left chest helps detect ETT migration into R mainstem.
- Risks: aspiration, gastric dilatation, respiratory compromise with positive-pressure ventilation

ANESTHETIC PLAN
- If medically unstable, gastrostomy before induction to relieve gastric distention
- Preoxygenation & suctioning of esophageal pouch before induction
- Consider awake intubation.
- Stable pts may have IV induction.
- Mask induction can be performed, but positive-pressure ventilation should be minimized or avoided until ligation of fistula.
- Proper positioning of ETT achieved by placing into R mainstem & withdrawing until breath sounds heard at L axilla. Alternatively, the fistula can be isolated by passing a 3 Fr Fogarty into the fistula track.
- Gastric distention can occur, resulting in resp compromise & CV collapse requiring emergency gastrostomy.
- Maintenance: after TEF ligation, balanced technique with NMB & controlled ventilation
- Risks: hypoxemia from R lung compression, kinking of bronchus, or blood in the trachea and endotracheal tube
- Emergence: extubation usually deferred until stable in NICU

PAIN MANAGEMENT
- Systemic: titrate IV opioids
- Regional: caudal catheter threaded to thoracic level: use 2% lidocaine, 3% 2-chloroprocaine, 0.1-0.2% ropivacaine or 0.125% bupivacaine intraop

PACU/POSTOPERATIVE CONSIDERATIONS
- Orogastric tube marked to level of esophageal anastomosis
- Epidural analgesia with 2% 2-chloroprocaine, 1.5% lidocaine, 0.1% ropivacaine or 0.0625-0.125% bupivacaine
- Avoid head extension: puts tension on anastomosis
- Complications: anastomotic leak, tracheo- or bronchomalacia & pneumothorax

---

TRACHEOSTOMY

ORIGINALLY WRITTEN BY ABBOY MOHAN, MD
REVISED BY RONALD S. LITMAN, DO

CO-EXISTING DISEASES
- Chronically intubated pts with respiratory insufficiency requiring mechanical ventilation & PEEP
- Can be performed in ICU if special ventilatory requirements
- Upper airway obstruction (eg, Ludwig's angina, pharyngeal abscess)

PREOPERATIVE ASSESSMENT
- Recent ABG & CXR
- Other labs as indicated
- Premed: titrate midazolam
- NPO: std

PROCEDURAL CONSIDERATIONS
- Supine with shoulder roll & neck extension
- Pts either have ETT in place or trach is performed for upper airway obstruction in unintubated pt.
- ETT should be accessible to be moved proximal to trach site.
- Do not remove ETT from airway so it can be pushed back into distal trachea if there is difficulty with trach insertion.
- IV fluids: LR or equiv

- Monitors: std
- Risks: pneumothorax, hemorrhage, aspiration of blood, pneumomediastinum, difficult trach tube insertion
- Immediately after trach insertion, confirm position by auscultation & capnograph

ANESTHETIC PLAN

- IV or inhalation induction may be used in intubated pts
- For pts with airway compromise or anticipated difficult intubation, maintain spontaneous ventilation with local anesthesia or inhalation anesthesia with mask or LMA.
- Maintenance: inhalation agents, narcotics & NMBs may be used in intubated pts
- Emergence: child usually ventilated postop
- Adjuvant tx: bronchodilator

PAIN MANAGEMENT

- Systemic: titrate intraop opioid of choice
- Regional: local anesthetic before tracheostomy

PACU/POSTOPERATIVE CONSIDERATIONS

- Analgesia: titrate opioids if not ventilated
- CXR to confirm proper trach placement & R/O pneumothorax or pneumomediastinum
- Recurrent laryngeal nerve damage & hematoma may cause airway compromise

---

TYMPANOMASTOIDECTOMY

PAUL TRIPI, MD

CO-EXISTING DISEASES

- Chronic middle ear disease, cholesteatoma
- Can have hearing loss

PREOPERATIVE ASSESSMENT
- Studies: none
- Premed: midazolam
- NPO: std

PROCEDURAL CONSIDERATIONS
- Supine with head lateral
- OR table turned 90–180°
- Drapes cover head & neck, difficult access to airway
- IV fluids: LR
- One IV adequate to replace fasting deficit & maint fluids
- Min blood & 3rd space fluid loss
- Monitors: std & visual monitoring of facial movement if requested by surgeon
- Consider Foley if >3 h
- Risks: performed using a microscope; need pt immobile & min bleeding
- Surgeon may request no NMBs so facial nerve can be monitored.
- Changes in middle ear pressure & volume must be avoided if tympanic graft placed at end of procedure.
- Hyperthermia due to complete coverage by surgical drapes

ANESTHETIC PLAN
- Standard inhalation induction with sevoflurane, or IV induction with agent of choice
- NMB may be used to facilitate Intubation.
- Long-acting NMBs should be avoided if surgeon wants facial nerve monitoring.
- Alternatively, pt can be intubated under deep anesthesia without NMB.
- ETT required
- Maintenance: balanced technique: O_2, N_2O & volatile agent
- Use of N_2O should be discussed with surgeon, who may request that it be discontinued before placement of tympanic graft

- Emergence: surgeon may request deep extubation
- Adjuvant tx: antiemetic (eg, ondansetron) for PONV

PAIN MANAGEMENT

- Systemic: small amounts of opioid to supplement GA and provide preemptive analgesia
- Regional: subQ infiltration of local anesthesia by surgeon

PACU/POSTOPERATIVE CONSIDERATIONS

- Nausea/vomiting common
- Pt may have difficulty with hearing & equilibrium.
- Pain is mild to moderate.
- Mild analgesics (eg, acetaminophen, ibuprofen) may be adequate.
- IV morphine sometimes necessary
- If pain and nausea under control, some pts may be discharged home.

UMBILICAL HERNIA REPAIR

ANTHONY M. FERNANDEZ, DO AND ZEEV N. KAIN, MD

CO-EXISTING DISEASES

- Hypothyroidism or thyroid dysgenesis
- Chromosomal abnormalities:
  - ➤ Trisomy 13 & 18
  - ➤ Hurler's syndrome
  - ➤ Beckwith-Wiedemann syndrome
  - ➤ Rare complications include incarceration, strangulation & perforation.

PREOPERATIVE ASSESSMENT

- Studies: none
- Premed: if > 1 yr, PO midazolam 0.5 mg/kg; max 15 mg, Tylenol 10–20 mg/kg
- NPO: std

PROCEDURAL CONSIDERATIONS

■ Supine
■ IV fluids: LR maintenance; 3rd space loss minimal: 0–2 mL/kg/h
■ Minimal blood loss
■ Monitors: std

ANESTHETIC PLAN

■ Inhalation induction with sevoflurane or IV induction with agent of choice
■ Endotracheal intubation, mask or LMA all OK
■ Maintenance: $N_2O + O_2$ + volatile agent or TIVA
■ Opioids titrated as needed
■ Surgeon may request paralysis
■ Awaken & extubate in OR

PAIN MANAGEMENT

■ Intraop opioid of choice
■ Regional (rectus sheath block) or local infiltration by surgeon

PACU / POSTOPERATIVE CONSIDERATIONS

■ Treat PONV with ondansetron or metoclopramide.
■ Analgesia: acetaminophen or ibuprofen

URETERAL REIMPLANT

PASQUALE DE NEGRI, MD

CO-EXISTING DISEASES

■ Congenital vesicoureteral reflux
■ Hydronephrosis; chronic UTI
■ Renal failure; hypertension

PREOPERATIVE ASSESSMENT

■ Studies: lytes, creatinine only if renal damage present
■ Premed: if >1 yr, PO midazolam 0.5 mg/kg; max 15 mg

- NPO: std

PROCEDURAL CONSIDERATIONS
- Supine usually
- IV fluids: warmed LR; 3rd space loss 6–10 mL/kg/h
- Maintain euvolemia to facilitate postop urine flow & avoid clots
- Monitors: std
- Risks: hypothermia; use forced warm air blanket underneath & around pt & HME in breathing circuit

ANESTHETIC PLAN
- Inhalation induction with sevoflurane or IV induction with propofol or thiopental
- NMB of choice to facilitate intubation & surgical access
- Maintenance: balanced technique: O_2, air, volatile agent
- Awaken & extubate in OR

PAIN MANAGEMENT
- Systemic: titrate fentanyl or alfentanil intraop
- Regional: continuous epidural using 1% lidocaine, 0.25% bupivacaine or 0.2% ropivacaine or 0.25% levobupivacaine

PACU/POSTOPERATIVE CONSIDERATIONS
- Analgesia: if epidural present, continuous infusion: 0.0625–0.125% levobupivacaine (max 0.25 mg/kg/h) or 0.1% ropivacaine + opioid or clonidine 2 mcg/kg at outset of infusion
- Systemic: PO acetaminophen with codeine, or IV morphine 0.05–0.1 mg/kg prn or PCA in appropriate pts

---

VASCULAR RING REPAIR

CHARLIZE KESSIN, MD

CO-EXISTING DISEASES
- Tracheal and/or esophageal compression

- Wheezing, stridor, coughing, difficulty feeding, cardio-respiratory arrest 5 causes:
- Double aortic arch (45–65%)
- R aortic arch with L ligamentum arteriosum
- Anomalous innominate a
- Anomalous L carotid a
- Anomalous L pulmonary a (partial vascular ring or pulmonary sling)
- Assoc with congenital heart disease
- Resp failure: chronic infection, vascular compression resulting in emphysema that compresses other lung tissue
- If airway compression at carina or main bronchus, a normally situated ETT will not relieve obstruction.
- May need endotracheal intubation preop to relieve serious symptoms
- Air trapping in a lobe from vascular compression alleviated by application of PEEP

PREOPERATIVE ASSESSMENT
- Studies: none
- Premed: if >1 yr, PO midazolam 0.5 mg/kg; max 15 mg
- NPO: std

PROCEDURAL CONSIDERATIONS
- Prone for median sternotomy or lateral for posterolateral thoracotomy or video-assisted thoracoscopy
- IV fluids: LR via large-bore IV
- Anticipate uncontrolled bleed
- Monitors: std with two pulse oximeters + A-line for pulmonary artery sling +/− cerebral oximetry for anastomosis near the carotid artery
- Esophageal steth can cause airway obstruction.
- Risks: bleeding, airway obstruction, hypoxemia from lung compression

- Complications: tracheomalacia, chylothorax & diaphragmatic paralysis

ANESTHETIC PLAN

- Airway obstruction is main concern.
- Insert ETT past site of tracheal compression; may need long ETT with side holes to ventilate other bronchus, or ventilate via bronchoscope.
- Induction: no preferences; avoid NMB until airway controlled
- Maintenance: balanced technique: volatile agent, O_2 & air
- Emergence: postop intubation required if traumatic intubation or tracheomalacia present
- Adjuvant tx: lidocaine before inserting bronchoscope into distal airway

PAIN MANAGEMENT

- Systemic: titrate opioids; morphine or fentanyl preferred
- Regional: thoracic epidural catheter via caudal canal after induction & intubation

PACU/POSTOPERATIVE CONSIDERATIONS

- Analgesia: if epidural catheter (pt >1 yr) 0.1% bupivacaine or 0.15% ropivacaine +/– fentanyl 0.02 mcg/mL or +/– clonidine 0.4 mcg/mL bolus of 0.1–0.2 mL/kg prn or if PCEA: infusion rate of 0.1 mL/kg/h, bolus of 0.1 mL/kg, lockout of 20 min, total infusion in 1 h 0.2–0.4 mL/kg
- Systemic: IV morphine 50 mcg/kg over 10 min prn; or if PCA: infusion rate of 20 mcg/kg/h, bolus of 20 mcg/kg, lockout 10 min, total in 1 h 100 mcg/kg
- Humidified O_2
- Respiratory physiotherapy
- Epinephrine or dexamethasone if airway swelling
- Extubate when edema & tracheomalacia absent

VENTRICULAR SEPTAL DEFECT REPAIR

STEPHEN A. STAYER, MD

CO-EXISTING DISEASES
- Associated heart lesions: PDA, ASD, PS, subaortic stenosis, coarc of aorta
- CHF related to the degree of L to R shunt proportional to size of VSD
- Tx: digoxin, diuretics and/or ACE inhibitors

PREOPERATIVE ASSESSMENT
- Studies: ECG, CXR, echo, CBC, lytes, BUN, creat, coags
- Cardiac cath usually not necessary
- Premed: if >1 yr, PO midazolam 0.5 mg/kg; max 15 mg
- NPO: std

PROCEDURAL CONSIDERATIONS
- Supine
- IV fluids: balanced salt solution: (LR, Plasmalyte, Normosol) + glucose for infants
- Minimize IV fluids before CPB
- 5% albumin for volume bolus will limit total fluids & maintain colloid osmotic pressure.
- IV fluids, PRBC, FFP warmed
- Monitors: std + A-line, CVP, Foley
- TEE std in many centers
- Neuro: BIS, cerebral oximeter, transcranial Doppler used in some centers
- Transfusion common in pts <10 kg
- Risks: major neuro m/m <1% in large centers; air embolism minimized with use of TEE; low cardiac output due to myocardial injury or significant residual shunting; pulmonary htn; heart block

ANESTHETIC PLAN

- Inhalation or IV induction
- Avoid myocardial depressants (halothane, thiopental).
- Pts with significant CHF sensitive to inhalation agents
- Maintenance: opioid-based, fentanyl or sufentanil with low doses of isoflurane or midazolam
- Avoid N_2O: air embolism & increasing size of microbubbles
- Emergence: pts with good LV fn extubated in OR or immed postop
- Pts with limited myocardial reserve should remain intubated & ventilated in ICU.
- Adjuvant tx: inotropic agents (epinephrine) readily available for low cardiac output
- Occasional pt will require epicardial pacing.
- Rarely NO used to tx pulmonary htn

PAIN MANAGEMENT

- Systemic: fentanyl or sufentanil
- Regional: caudal epidural, spinal or thoracic epidural opioids & local anesthetics. However, controversial because of systemic heparinization

PACU/POSTOPERATIVE CONSIDERATIONS

- Analgesia: morphine most common via intermittent dosing, continuous infusion or PCA
- Same risks as intraop

VIDEO-ASSISTED THORACOSCOPIC SURGERY (VATS)

RONALD S. LITMAN, DO

CO-EXISTING DISEASES

- Depends on indications: empyema, pneumonia, interstitial lung disease, metastases, congenital lung malformations

PREOPERATIVE ASSESSMENT

- Studies: hct, T&S
- Premed: if >1 yr, PO midazolam 0.5 mg/kg; max 10 mg
- NPO: std

PROCEDURAL CONSIDERATIONS

- Position: lat decub
- IV fluids: warmed LR; 3rd space loss 5-10 mL/kg/h
- Monitors: std + A-line if significant pulmonary disease
- Usually need OLV for lung isolation
- OLV in infants commonly causes hypoxemia; may need to reinflate lung occasionally during procedure
- Smallest DLT 26F: outer diameter 87 mm, same as 6.5 ETT; use for pts >7–8 yr
- Univent tube: self-contained bronchial blocker; smallest tube has 35-mm uncuffed blocker: has 80-mm outer diameter; comparable to 5.5 ID tube (for pts >6 yr)
- Methods for OLV in pts <7–8 yr: mainstem intubation of non-operative side with normal ETT; advance until breath sounds on contralateral side disappear; facilitate by turning pt's head to contralateral side while advancing tube with bevel facing contralateral side; cuff may cause obstruction of RUL bronchus; use fiberoptic bronchoscope for initial placement or confirmation
- Bronchial blockade with Fogarty balloon catheter: <2 yr use 4F; >2 yr use 5F; can't suction or give CPAP
- Foley catheter into bronchus
- Pulmonary artery catheter with balloon into bronchus
- Always confirm bronchial intubation with fiberoptic bronchoscopy
- Risks: damage to mainstem bronchus from bronchial blocker; herniation of bronchial blocker cuff into trachea; failure to obtain adequate bronchial seal; hypoxemia from shunt through nonventilated lung

ANESTHETIC PLAN

- Induction: IV or volatile agent of choice, NMB of choice
- Maintenance: balanced technique: O_2, air, volatile agent; avoid N_2O
- Unless significant lung disease, awaken & extubate in OR

PAIN MANAGEMENT

- Systemic: titrate opioid intraop
- Regional: intercostal blocks; epidural if expect significant postop pain

PACU/POSTOPERATIVE CONSIDERATIONS

- Analgesia: if epidural present continue local anesthetic and/or opioid
- IV morphine 0.05 mg/kg prn

VOLVULUS (MALROTATION)

SEMYON FISHKIN, MD

CO-EXISTING DISEASES

- Intestinal malrotation, polysplenia, asplenia, congenital abdominal wall defects, pyloric stenosis, esophageal atresia, ileal/jejunal atresia or duplication, biliary atresia, duodenal web/atresia, Meckel's diverticulum, Down syndrome, trisomy 13/18, diaphragmatic hernia, VACTERL association, situs inversus and asplenia, congenital heart disease, renal anomalies, cystic fibrosis, Hirschprung disease, gastric volvulus, agenesis of corpus callosum.

PREOPERATIVE ASSESSMENT

- Studies: hct; others defined by coexisting diseases and medical status (e.g., electrolytes, coagulation tests, blood glucose, blood gas, ECHO)
- Premed: none

- NPO: full stomach
- Volume status assessment

PROCEDURAL CONSIDERATIONS
- Supine
- IV fluids: normal saline or LR (if no hyperkalemia) plus maintenance with dextrose-containing solution if neonate/infant
- Consider colloid if large fluid requirements
- Monitors: std. + Foley; A-line, CVP if clinically indicated
- Bleeding usually minimal unless pt coagulopathic
- Risks: increased intraabdominal pressure due to bowel edema during abdominal closure
- Hypothermia: warm IV fluids, forced warm air blanket, increase OR temp

ANESTHETIC PLAN
- Consider fluid bolus with re-assessment before induction if hypovolemic
- Induction: RSI with sux (if no contraindications) or rocuronium
- ETT required
- Maintenance: O_2, air, volatile agent
- Premature babies and sick neonates may not tolerate potent halogenated agents.
- GI decompression: OG or NG tube
- Consider leaving intubated if premature, septic/unstable, extensive bowel resection or "2nd look" planned.
- Consider inotropic support
- Perioperative antibiotics
- Management of co-existing conditions

PAIN MANAGEMENT
- Systemic: titrate fentanyl/morphine
- Regional: consider epidural via caudal, lumbar or low thoracic route

POSTOPERATIVE CONSIDERATIONS

- Correct hypovolemia if present
- Continue epidural analgesia if present; otherwise IV opioids
- Avoid epidural opioids if pt <1 yr

V-P SHUNT INSERTION/REVISION

JOEL O. JOHNSON, MD, PhD AND JOSEPH D. TOBIAS, MD

CO-EXISTING DISEASES

- If congenital hydrocephalus: look for other defects
- Acquired hydrocephalus: IVH in preemies
- Tumors
- Signs & symp: lethargy, vomiting, altered mental status, downward gaze

PREOPERATIVE ASSESSMENT

- Lytes if vomiting
- Check hydration
- Check for increased ICP
- No premed if ICP increased
- Premeds: GI prophylaxis prn
- If >1 yr, PO midazolam 0.5 mg/kg; max 15 mg in acetaminophen 10–15 mg/kg; or IV midazolam: 0.03–0.05 mg/kg
- NPO: std

PROCEDURAL CONSIDERATIONS

- Position: supine, bed turned 90°
- IV fluids: LR; replace deficit, maintenance & 3rd space losses 2–3 mL/kg/h
- Glucose for pts with inadequate metabolic reserve
- Hyperglycemia may worsen neurologic injury.
- Monitors: std
- Risks: hypothermia with global CNS dysfunction

- V-pleural shunts–may require one lung ventilation
- V-atrial shunts–air embolism

ANESTHETIC PLAN
- IV induction for pts with increased ICP & adults
- Thiopental, etomidate or propofol, nondepolarizing NMB
- Cricoid pressure
- Inhalation: sevoflurane
- Halothane OK if hyperventilation initiated ASAP
- Cricoid pressure & modified RSI, placement of IV ASAP
- Hyperventilation before intubation
- Maintenance: balanced technique with fentanyl 2–3 mcg/kg up front
- Avoid N_2O: may inc ICP & CBF
- Avoid hypotension: decreases CPP
- NMB not required unless entry into abdomen difficult
- Short-acting drugs (desflurane, sevoflurane, remifentanil) facilitate awakening.
- Avoid opioids at end of procedure.
- Awaken & extubate in OR
- Adjuvant tx: mannitol 0.25–0.5 g/kg
- Use only if symptomatic.

PAIN MANAGEMENT
- Low-dose opioid and/or PR acetaminophen 40 mg/kg
- NSAIDs contraindicated (bleeding)
- Local anesthetic infiltration

PACU/POSTOPERATIVE CONSIDERATIONS
- Acetaminophen or low-dose opioid
- Avoid CNS depression.
- Observe for airway obstruction & change in neuro status.
- If obtunded: consider shunt malfunction/intracranial bleed: get emergent CT

WILMS' TUMOR EXCISION

DAVID A. YOUNG, MD, FAAP

CO-EXISTING DISEASES
- Bilateral in 5%, painless mass
- Abdominal pain; fever; hematuria
- Hypertension; GI symptoms
- Acquired Von Willebrand's disease
- Chemotx toxicity: cardiomyopathy with doxorubicin (Adriamycin)
- Radiation tx if lung mets

PREOPERATIVE ASSESSMENT
- Studies: CBC, BUN, creat, LFTs, coags, T&C
- Radiology: size/location of mass; assess for extension into IVC/right atrium
- MUGA or ECHO if prior doxorubicin
- CXR if prior rad tx; echo if atrium involved
- Premed: midazolam, consider ranitidine/metoclopramide
- NPO: std

PROCEDURAL CONSIDERATIONS
- Contralateral exploration & nephrectomy
- Supine
- IV fluids: LR; bleeding variable
- Possibility of massive blood loss especially if IVC involved
- Large-bore IV × 2 in upper extremity and/or neck
- Blood products in OR
- 3rd space loss > 10 mL/kg/hr
- Arterial/central line based on size/location of mass & preop cardiorespiratory status
- Risks: sudden massive hemorrhage, embolism, hypotension from IVC compression

ANESTHETIC PLAN

- RSI + cricoid pressure if full stomach; otherwise inhalational induction with agent of choice
- Maintenance: balanced technique: volatile agent, opioid, NMB
- Awaken & extubate in OR if hemodynamically stable

PAIN MANAGEMENT

- Systemic: titrate IV opioid
- Regional: epidural: caudal/lumbar
- Most placed under GA; caudal for age <5
- Dose after hemostasis achieved: 0.1–0.25% bupivacaine or 0.1–0.2% ropivacaine w/epi 1:200K
- 0.05 mL/kg/segment, max 1 mL/kg

PACU/POSTOPERATIVE CONSIDERATIONS

- Continuous epidural infusions: 0.0625–0.1% bupivacaine or 0.1% ropivacaine w/ fentanyl 2 mcg/mL or hydromorphone 10 mcg/mL or morphine 0.1 mg/mL: run at 0.1–0.4 mL/kg/hr
- Monitor volume status: oliguria from hypovolemia (bleeding) vs. compromised renal function
- Pain leads to splinting, atelectasis & hypoxemia.

PART THREE

Regional Anesthesia

EPIDURAL ANALGESIA

ARJUNAN GANESH, MBBS

INDICATIONS

- Postop: thoracotomy, laparotomy, procedures on hips and lower extremities
- Acute: chest & lower extremity trauma, sickle cell crisis
- Chronic: regional pain syndrome of lower extremities, pain from malignancy

PRE-PROCEDURAL ASSESSMENT

- Contraindications: history of bleeding disorder, spine abnormalities, previous spine surgery
- Informed consent
- Check for kyphoscoliosis or infection at sight of intended epidural placement.
- Detailed neurological exam to detect preexisting neuro deficits

PROCEDURAL MANAGEMENT

- Usually performed under general anesthesia in lateral decubitus position with adequate monitoring; if awake, sitting position may be used
- Caudal approach in neonate and young infants; direct lumbar or thoracic puncture in older children
- Sterile prep and drape; operator wears sterile gloves, hat and mask
- Tuohy or Crawford needle, loss of resistance to saline or air
- Thread catheter 3–5 cm into epidural space.
- Aspirate for CSF or blood, administer test dose: lidocaine with epinephrine 0.1 mL/kg (max 3 mL) to rule out intravascular/intrathecal placement. Look for T wave amplitude elevation, tachycardia, hypertension, lower extremity weakness (conscious pts).

- Start epidural infusion in OR. Bolus prior to infusion. Supplement with IV opioids as needed.
- Children <8 yrs rarely develop hypotension; treat with fluids and/or vasopressors.

POST-PROCEDURAL CONCERNS
- Examine pt for adequacy of sensory block, particularly if complaining of pain.
- Bolus with or without increasing hourly infusion rate may be used to improve analgesia.
- Monitor cardiorespiratory parameters and pain scores on regular schedule.
- If epidural opioids: use systemic opioids cautiously under adequate supervision.
- Treat nausea/vomiting with ondansetron/metoclopramide, pruritus with nalbuphine.
- If no urinary catheter, monitor for urinary retention.
- Inspect epidural catheter site at least every 24 hours; consider removing catheter if fever without obvious reasons.
- If worsening neurological deficit, consider epidural hematoma or abscess.

SPINAL ANESTHESIA

ARJUNAN GANESH, MBBS

INDICATIONS
- Procedures lasting <2 hrs below T10 dermatome
- Useful for former preemies <60 weeks post-conceptual age and full-term neonates at risk for postop apnea
- Useful for MH-susceptible pts, muscle biopsy procedure

PRE-PROCEDURAL ASSESSMENT
- Contraindications: history of bleeding disorder, spine abnormalities, previous spine surgery

- Informed consent
- Examine for kyphoscoliosis or infection at sight of intended placement.
- Detailed neuro exam to detect preexisting deficits

INTRAOPERATIVE MANAGEMENT
- Position: sitting or lateral decubitus
- Sterile prep and drape; operator wears sterile gloves, hat and mask
- 25G Whitacre needle with or without introducer; 22G Quincke used in neonates
- Local anesthetics: tetracaine 1%, bupivacaine 0.5% or 0.75%. Dextrose or epi may be added. Opioids may be added for postop analgesia.
- Carefully position pt after injection, particularly if hyperbaric solutions used; avoid leg elevation.
- Neonates and young children develop respiratory difficulties more than cardiovascular instability: autonomic nervous systems are not well developed.
- Monitor: BP, pulse oximetry, ECG
- Distracters if awake: pacifiers dipped in sugar; books, video games, or movies in older children
- If postop apnea not a concern, sedate with midazolam, N_2O, or propofol.
- Support BP with fluids.

POST-PROCEDURAL CONCERNS
- Examine for reversal of spinal blockade.
- Monitor cardiorespiratory parameters closely until block has worn off.
- If spinal opioid administered, continue monitoring until effect wears off.
- Monitor for urinary retention.
- Pts may experience transient neurological symptoms and will need reassurance and follow-up.

Printed in the United States
By Bookmasters